Super Simple Recipes for
WEIGHT-LOSS SURGERY RECOVERY

Quarto.com

© 2025 Quarto Publishing Group USA Inc.
Text © 2006 Margaret M. Furtado and Lynette Schultz

First Published in 2025 by New Shoe Press, an imprint of The Quarto Group,
100 Cummings Center, Suite 265-D, Beverly, MA 01915, USA.
T (978) 282-9590 F (978) 283-2742

Essential, In-Demand Topics, Four-Color Design, Affordable Price

New Shoe Press publishes affordable, beautifully designed books covering evergreen, in-demand subjects. With a goal to inform and inspire readers' everyday hobbies, from cooking and gardening to wellness and health to art and crafts, New Shoe titles offer the ultimate library of purposeful, how-to guidance aimed at meeting the unique needs of each reader. Reimagined and redesigned from Quarto's best-selling backlist, New Shoe books provide practical knowledge and opportunities for all DIY enthusiasts to enrich and enjoy their lives.

Visit Quarto.com/New-Shoe-Press for a complete listing of the New Shoe Press books.

New Shoe Press titles are also available at discount for retail, wholesale, promotional, and bulk purchase. For details, contact the Special Sales Manager by email at specialsales@quarto.com or by mail at The Quarto Group, Attn: Special Sales Manager, 100 Cummings Center, Suite 265-D, Beverly, MA 01915, USA.

10 9 8 7 6 5 4 3 2 1

ISBN: 978-0-7603-9090-0
eISBN: 978-0-7603-9091-7

The content in this book was previously published in *Recipes for Life After Weight-Loss Surgery* (Fair Winds Press 2007) by Margaret M. Furtado and Lynette Schultz.

Library of Congress Cataloging-in-Publication Data available

Photography: Steve Galvin

The information in this book is for educational purposes only. It is not intended to replace the advice of a physician or medical practitioner. Please see your health-care provider before beginning any new health program.

Printed in China

Super Simple Recipes for
WEIGHT-LOSS SURGERY RECOVERY

Easy, Delicious Recipes to Support Health

MARGARET M. FURTADO, MS, RD, LDN

LYNETTE SHULTZ, LRCP, RT

CHEF JOSEPH EWING, BS

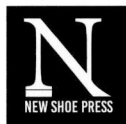

NEW SHOE PRESS

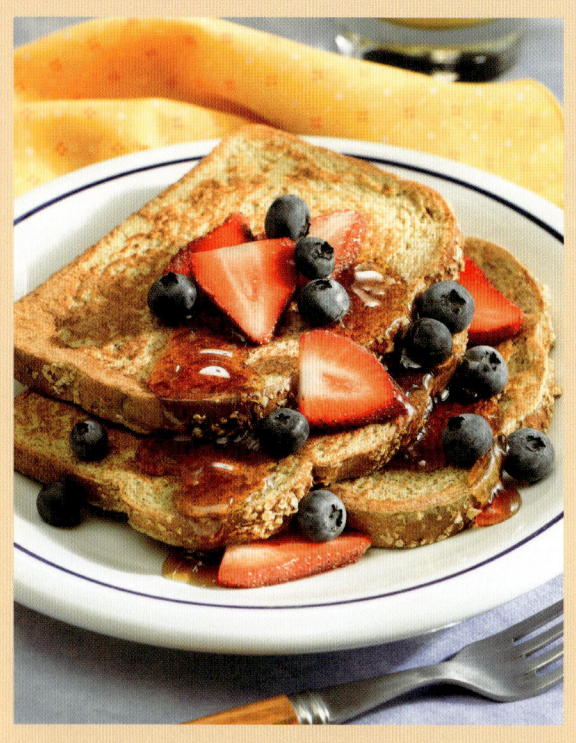

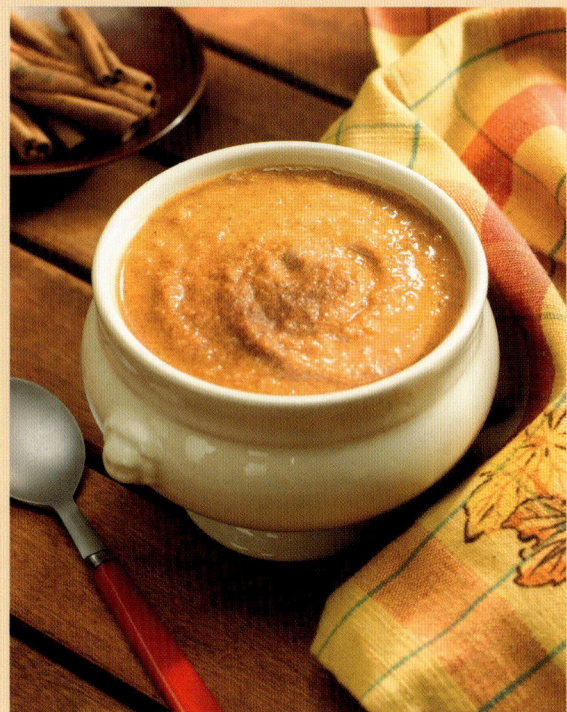

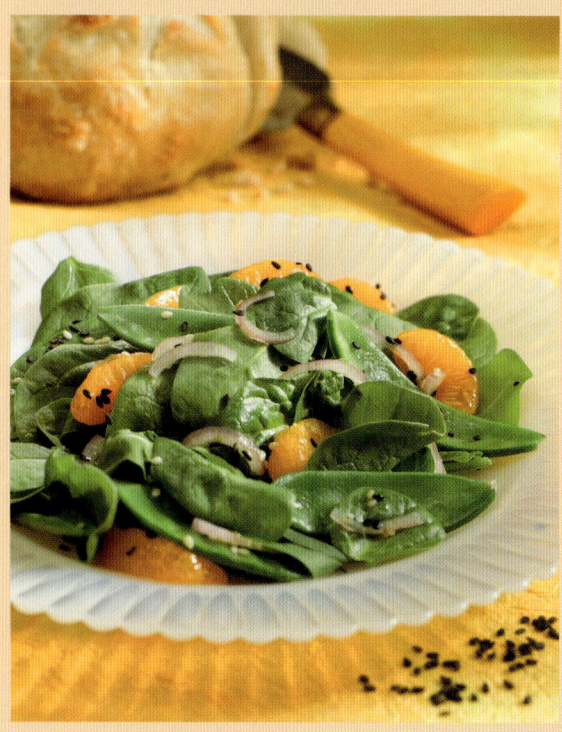

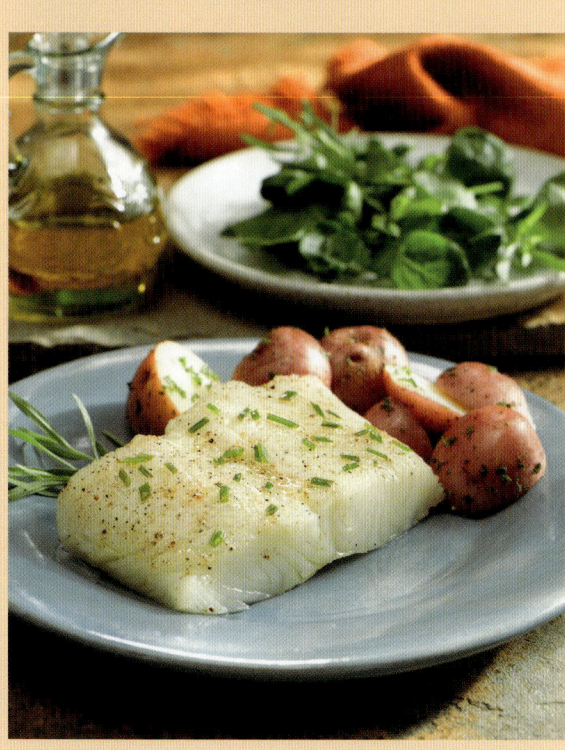

Contents

Introduction

Congratulations! You've made a very important decision to improve your health by having weight-loss surgery. Now it's time to use good nutrition to maximize not only your weight loss, but your health, vitality, and renewed sense of well-being. I'm happy to share my extensive nutrition background and expertise in weight-loss surgery with you, and I am thrilled you've chosen Super Simple Recipes for Weight-Loss Surgery Recovery *to help guide you in this exciting new period in your life! Let's get started!*

The guidelines outlined in the following pages are general instructions and suggestions that I typically provide to my bariatric surgery patients based upon years of experience and input from three different bariatric surgery centers of excellence I've had the privilege of working at. *Super Simple Recipes for Weight-Loss Surgery Recovery* features an amazing and well-trained chef, Joseph Ewing, B.S., with whom I had the pleasure to work on my second book. Joe is also a nutritionist, so he lends a great touch to the updated version of this book!

Also in this edition, I've included nutritional guidelines for a newly available and increasingly popular bariatric surgery called the vertical sleeve gastrectomy (VSG), commonly referred to as "the sleeve." I'm delighted to contribute my expertise here for the benefit of those who are either pursuing or already have had this excellent procedure; this information will also be handy for your loved ones and supporters.

The specific nutrition recommendations—such as calories, protein, vitamins, and minerals—are based upon the most recent research studies. However, because bariatric, or weight-loss, surgery is still a fairly new field, there may be variability among medical institutions and/or bariatric surgery teams, in terms of nutritional recommendations. Please check with your hospital's staff, including your dietitian, for your particular nutritional instructions.

The information provided in this section is general, rather than the exact diet I provide to my patients, because this book is meant to focus on our healthy recipes after your weight-loss surgery. I offer just an overview of clinical nutrition guidelines, such as foods that you may want to avoid because of common intolerances and foods

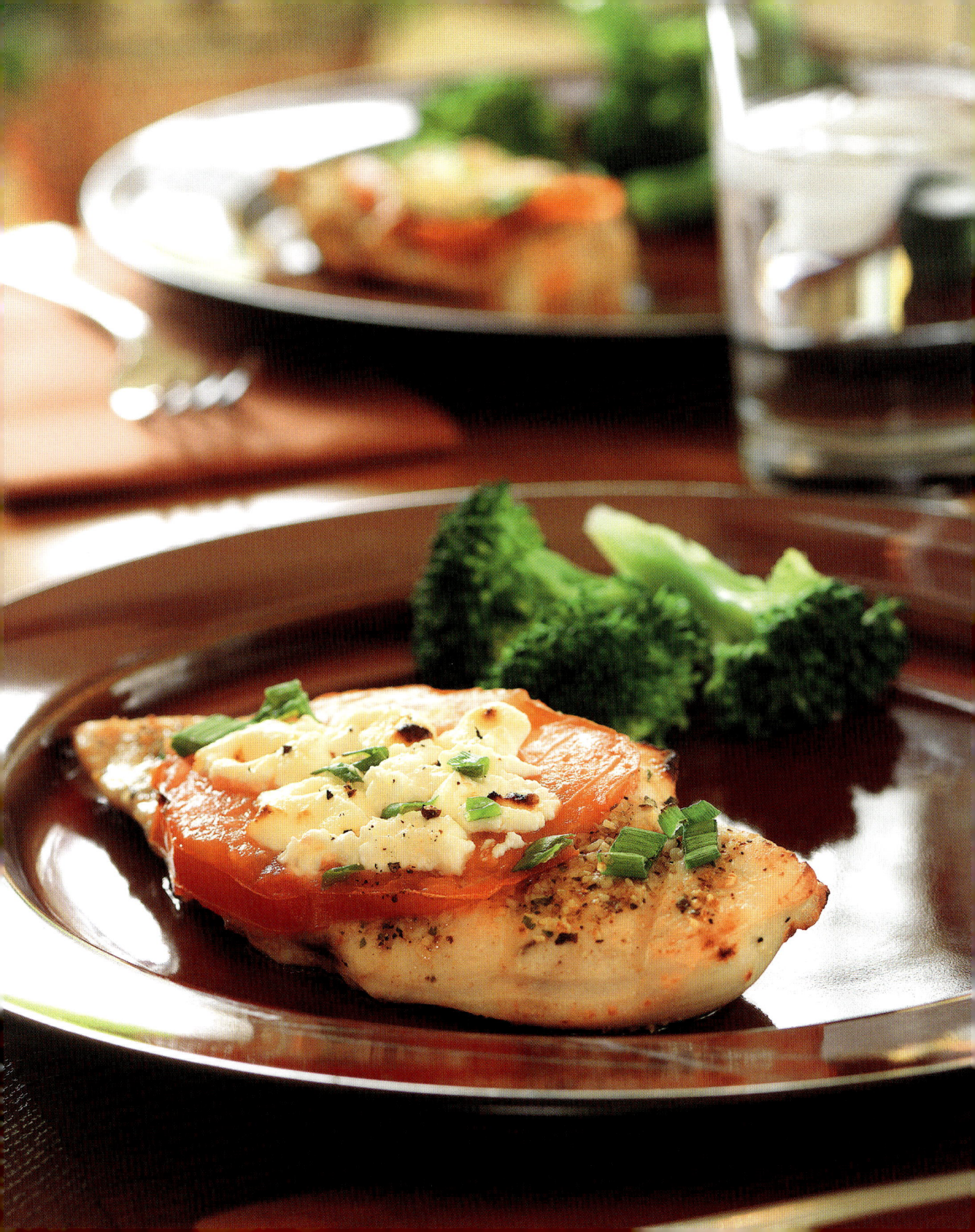

you may want to eat because of vitamins and minerals that may be deficient after your surgery.

Below each recipe title, you will see a texture category—Full Liquids, Puree, Mechanical Soft, or Regular—to help you decide when it might be appropriate to try that particular recipe. I've omitted the "weeks out" recommendation after each procedure, which was in the original version of this book, and replaced it with this classification of textures. I felt it would make the book easier to follow and would not contradict the suggested time frames provided by your surgical team for texture trials. I trust this will help streamline things for you and make it that much easier to navigate the "nutritional waters" after the often-times overwhelming initial weeks following your weight-loss surgery.

You should always keep in mind that your individual surgical center, as well as your individual tolerances, are key in terms of when you are ready to advance your diet and the foods your body can tolerate. Please listen to your body, as well as your surgical team members, and slowly add new foods as recommended, one new food at a time to better ascertain which food(s) your body is able to digest well. Keep in mind that these are merely suggestions and check with your center's dietitian and team for your specific diet guidelines.

Each recipe has been carefully analyzed for its nutritional content. After each recipe, you'll find the number of calories; grams of protein and carbohydrates; total fat, saturated fat, sugars, and fiber; and milligrams of cholesterol and sodium, for each serving. The nutritional analysis includes all ingredients in the recipe, except ingredients that are optional or garnishes, or the recipes for the rubs.

As you read these guidelines, and later on the recipes, please keep in mind that everyone is different and the recommendations in this book are just suggestions. You should always refer to your doctor and weight-loss surgery team for individual guidance regarding your diet, vitamins, etc. For example, your center might recommend that you puree all of your solid foods in a blender the first weeks or even a month or more after your weight-loss surgery. Many surgical centers have different philosophies regarding advancing the diet. As you get to the recipes in this book, you will notice that each is labeled with different textures, which will correspond with what stage you are at in your diet after surgery. The texture labels in the book are Full Liquids, Puree, Mechanical Soft, and regular (listed here in order from easiest tolerated to more advanced). As your diet progresses, you can choose recipes with textures that your doctor and dietitian have allowed as well as the food textures below that level (i.e., if you can tolerate a Mechanical Soft texture, you can also try the recipes labeled "Puree" and "Full Liquids." Please follow your center's diet instructions. You might need to wait a month or two before trying some of our recipes, but you'll get there when you're ready!

As you try the recipes, listen to your body and avoid foods that seem to be ill-tolerated (such as those that cause vomiting or chest pain). On the other hand, although many of my weight-loss surgery patients don't tolerate certain foods— such as doughy breads, rolls, pasta, and rice—you may find that you have no problem with them at all. However, the guidelines are based upon a solid nutritional foundation and general feedback from my weight-loss surgery patients regarding foods they often find hard to tolerate and those that seem to cause no problems at all. The recipes in this book were chosen based upon what most of my patients said they could tolerate. For example, I didn't think many weight-loss surgery patients could tolerate muffins, and I often discourage the doughy, high-calorie variety you might find at your local coffee shop. However, after requests from some of my surgical patients and a conference with my chef friend and coauthor, Lynette, nondoughy, healthy, tasty muffin recipes were born!

Tolerance for foods and eating after weight-loss surgery varies from one person to another, regardless of which weight-loss surgery they had. Please don't feel anxious or concerned if you find you cannot tolerate foods with which most people have no problem. We are all unique, and therefore only you can decide what feels right in your body.

Healthy Diet Guidelines for All Weight-Loss Surgeries

Before I review the nutrition guidelines following surgery, it's important to discuss the components of a healthy diet and how it relates to your diet. The word "diet" often has some negative connotations, but here it simply refers to your new healthy eating plan. As you'll see from our recipes, healthy eating can be delicious and easy!

Fluids

It may be easy to overlook, but dehydration or suboptimal fluid intake is the most frequent commonality among patients that I see after weight-loss surgery. This is not surprising since much of the population only drinks fluids when they're thirsty, which means they're already at least a little dehydrated. I often advise my weight-loss surgery patients to aim for at least 48 ounces of total fluid per day, but preferably at least 64 ounces per day. Even then, I recommend gauging urine color (if dark yellow or concentrated, you probably need to drink more fluid). Also, if you feel dizzy when you stand or sit, or you pinch the skin on your knuckle and it takes longer to "bounce back" than it usually does, you probably need more fluid.

It's very important to drink fluids, especially after weight-loss surgery, to help flush out toxins and to help your body run efficiently overall. Every time you ingest protein, your kidneys need water to flush out the toxins from the protein.

Water is the fluid I most highly recommend to patients to drink. However, I sometimes hear from patients that water tastes "heavy" or "metallic" right after weight-loss surgery. If this is the case, adding lemon, lime, or diluting your favorite calorie-free (non-carbonated) beverage with the water may help. If it doesn't, then drink unsweetened or artificially sweetened teas or other drinks (non carbonated).

Juice can be dehydrating, and may even cause dumping syndrome (the sweaty, shaky, awful feeling some gastric bypass surgery patients get after eating sweets after surgery) if you drink them quickly and they're more concentrated. It's best to avoid juices altogether for weight loss, as well as overall tolerance. I don't advise more than 4 ounces of any kind of juice per day (especially not grape or cranberry juice, unless they're diet juices), since juice beverages are typically high in sugar and calories.

Caffeinated drinks like regular coffee and tea are typically discouraged, especially right after surgery, since caffeine is a diuretic and getting enough fluid in after surgery is difficult for a lot of people. Decaffeinated coffee or tea are fine, as long as you're not adding cream or sugar (skim milk or artificial sweeteners are okay).

Carbonated beverages are also generally discouraged because they tend to cause gas and bloating, which are already an issue for many people (at least for a brief period after surgery). In addition, there is a school of thought among some surgeons and other clinicians that continuous pressure from carbonated beverages could widen the connection from the new stomach pouch to the middle part of the small intestine (among gastric bypass patients), and this could lessen the feeling of fullness, which could cause weight regain, or lessen overall weight loss.

Alcohol after weight-loss surgery is generally discouraged, especially within the first six months, since it is a diuretic. Check with your doctor regarding alcohol; he or she will likely recommend that you have only a very small amount (if any).

In some of our recipes, you will find wine in the ingredient list, since it's often used for flavor. Even though the alcohol evaporates during the cooking process, substitutions for alcohol have

been provided. The flavor should be just as good, and the peace of mind of not worrying about having alcohol in the house will be priceless.

Possible challenges with fluids. Over the years, I've often heard from my patients that, other than the metallic taste, water "sits heavy" or "won't go down." What seems to help them, at least 99 percent of the time, is putting water or other liquids, including protein drinks, in the freezer. I've had patients go from only 20 ounces of fluid per day to more than 60 ounces by making just this change. Why would this work? Well, from chemistry refresher courses I recently took, ice is less dense than water—hence, why it floats—so the lower density of the ice helps it to go down better. Sugar-free popsicles might help, too, but I recommend adding them toward the end of the day rather than the beginning so that they won't take your appetite or, if you had gastric bypass surgery, room in your pouch.

If, however, you're constantly craving ice or waking up to chew on ice, talk to your surgical team immediately, because chronic or very strong ice cravings could very well be a red flag for iron deficiency, the most common issue long-term after gastric bypass surgery. (Studies reveal that 20 years after gastric bypass surgery, 50 percent of both men and nonmenstruating women may be low in iron.) Please keep in mind that dehydration is among the most common immediate issues after weight-loss surgery. If your urine is more apple juice–color than straw-color, speak to your surgical team, including your dietitian, right away. You don't want to end up back in the hospital one week after your surgery because you couldn't get enough fluids in!

Protein

Protein will always be important in your diet, both before and after your weight-loss surgery. Your surgical center will provide you with specific guidelines for protein intake, but I generally recommend a minimum of 60–80 grams of protein per day (before and after your surgery), and higher amounts if you've had BPD surgery (up to 120 grams of protein per day may be needed). As you'll see in the clinical nutrition guidelines in chapter 1, protein is very important for proper healing after surgery, as well as for life-long health. If you're not taking in enough protein, it could, in the long run, cause serious health problems, such as edema, or fluid build-up in the bodily tissue. Other protein deficiency-related health problems include anemia, as well as hair loss (which is often linked to rapid weight

loss rather than nutritional deficiencies, but could be worsened by low protein in the diet).

In the first weeks or months after surgery, your diet may be 40 to 50 percent protein due to lower food intake overall, and the inability to eat much at one time. This higher percentage of protein early on after your weight-loss surgery is recommended in order to help you meet your body's protein needs.

Foods high in protein include egg whites, meat, chicken, fish, tofu, and dairy products. As you'll read in the following chapters, meat and chicken, especially if dry or tough, may not go down well, so you will want to make sure these foods are moist and diced rather than grilled. Some people also have a problem with lactose intolerance after gastric bypass surgery, so if you experience this (gas, bloating, and diarrhea are possible signs), try substituting low-sugar soy milk or take a lactase enzyme pill with the milk products to help your body digest the milk sugar. Probiotics ("healthy bacteria"), such as acidophilus, might also help with lactose intolerance, since it may help your body better digest lactose, or milk sugar. Speak to your doctor or dietitian about whether probiotics may be for you after your surgery. There's so much research going on right now with probiotics, including the possibility of improving vitamin

B12 levels, as well as helping with constipation and overall gastrointestinal upset. Some research suggests these healthy bacteria might even help you maintain a healthy weight!

Carbohydrates

In this day of low-carb dieting, "carbohydrates" is almost a dirty word when it comes to diets. However, it's important for weight-loss surgery patients to incorporate healthy carbohydrates into their diets, both before and after surgery. Healthy carbs include 100 percent whole wheat bread (thin slices or toast are better tolerated than thick slices), brown rice, whole wheat pasta, and fresh fruit and vegetables. However, right after your weight loss surgery, you are typically not allowed to have these foods, since they're not well tolerated right away. Be sure to stick with foods recommended by your doctor during this time.

I generally recommend that most people include at least 40 percent of carbohydrates in their total caloric intake, both prior to surgery and for a few months after surgery, to provide energy. Carbohydrates are the premiere sources of energy for the brain and the body in general, so if you're not ingesting enough carbohydrates in the months after your surgery, you may very well find that your energy is lacking, to say the least. In this revised edition, I've included sample menus, for use both early postop and several months down the road, with suggested carbohydrate (and protein) levels to help your body function at its best. Don't be afraid of carbs! As I tell my patients: These days, the word "carb" is a dreaded, four-letter word. But carbohydrates help you get energy and they can help your body "spare" protein to ensure that the protein you take in is actually used for your muscles and to help you heal. My carbohydrate recommendations for my patients are 70 grams by 3 months out, 100 grams by 6 months out, and the Recommended Daily Allowance (RDA) of 130 grams by 1 year out. From my clinical experience, I'm convinced that patients who are able to reach these carbohydrate "milestones" have more energy, are better able to oxidize fat (the research confirms this), and, anecdotally, seem not only to lose more weight but have an easier time adapting to a maintenance diet of a healthy balance of fruits, vegetables, protein, and good fats.

Sugars

You'll notice in the recipes that I've included "sugars" information. Every 4 grams of "sugars" represents 1 teaspoon (or 1 packet) of sugar.

There are varying schools of thought, but dumping syndrome may increase if you're consuming foods or beverages high in simple sugars. The term "sugars" on a nutrition label refers to simple sugars. Even if you never "dump" or had the banding surgery, which does not involve dumping risk, it's still not a bad idea to watch the sugars in your diet. I've restricted the recipes to about 15 grams of sugars or less (no more than 4 teaspoons of sugar) for general health. Your surgical center may allow you more sugar than this, but I think you'll find the recipes just as delicious without the extra sugar.

Fats

In order to have a balanced, healthy diet, try to limit fats in your diet to no more than 30 percent of your total calories. Ideally, most of the fat in your diet will come from "heart-healthy" fats, such as olive, macadamia, and peanut oils. These fats will help decrease total cholesterol and low-density lipoproteins (LDLs). Heart-healthy fats may also have a role in increasing the good cholesterol, or high-density lipoproteins (HDLs). However, please keep in mind that even healthy fats are higher in calories compared to carbohydrates and proteins. In moderation, healthy fats can be part of a healthy, balanced diet, but try to keep the overall calories from fat no greater than 30 percent, even if they're healthy fats.

The least healthy fats of all are the trans fatty acids, followed by the saturated fats. Trans fats are typically found in processed foods, such as french fries, peanut butter, crackers, and margarine. Such fats are extremely unhealthy and raise levels of bad cholesterol, so try to avoid them. (Trans fats are formed by a process known as hydrogenation, which turns the fat into a solid and is used by food manufacturers to extend the shelf life of their products.) When you look at a food label's ingredients, trans fat can be spotted by the term "partially hydrogenated."

Saturated fats are hard at room temperature, and include stick butter and margarine, bacon, and fatty cuts of meat. Saturated fats are also included in the nutrition information, so please read all labels. After a while, you'll be a pro at deciphering which foods are the best health bargains, and to which ones you just want to say "no."

A Word about Calories

I can't tell you how often my patients ask me, "But Margaret, how many calories should I be eating?" While I respect that they want to look at calories, and may have counted calories all their lives, I try deemphasizing calories and instead focus on the proper nourishing of their bodies. For example, a healthy level of protein is 60 to 80 grams per day for most patients. Healthy levels of carbohydrates are those I noted on page 13. As for fat, if you're using online food logs that calculate fat grams, strive for somewhere between 20 and 50 grams of fat per day, depending, of course, on how far out from surgery you are and how much total food per day is appropriate for your body and level of physical activity.

Don't worry if you're not eating more than 500 or so calories in the first weeks, or even months, after your surgery. Studies show the "average" bariatric surgery patient doesn't consume more than 500 to 700 calories a day within the first few months of surgery. Your body will take what it needs from your fat reserves (sorry that there isn't a more eloquent way to put this!) and you'll be okay, as long as you get fluids, healthy carbohydrates (e.g., fruits, veggies, whole grains), your protein goal, and some healthy fats (as stated on the previous page). Of course, taking your vitamin/mineral supplements is also key to properly nourishing your body after your weight-loss procedure. Talk to your dietitian about supplements of calcium, and, if applicable, vitamin B12, iron, and (if you've had duodenal switch surgery) fat-soluble vitamins.

Remember, this is a new, healthy way of nourishing your body. Of course, if you find your weight is headed up fast, perhaps due to "dietary indiscretions," I highly recommend keeping careful food logs (paper or online), and bring the logs when you see your dietitian or surgical team member to better decipher why you're gaining weight. Some weight gain (5 pounds or so, on average) from your lowest weight after surgery is common and to be expected, but more than that, or rapid weight gain, should be brought to the immediate attention of your surgical team.

This deemphasis on calories is why you won't see listed the caloric content of most of our new meal plans. Rest assured, they're adequate for most people at the particular time points noted. If your center suggests a particular calorie level for you, however, it's not wrong, since every center does things differently. Calories are just not what I like to focus on.

Fiber

If you look at a food label, you'll see that fiber is actually included under carbohydrates in the nutrition information. However, by definition, humans do not possess the enzyme necessary to use fiber for calories or energy, which explains the recent trend to exclude fiber from the carbohydrate content of foods.

There are two kinds of fiber: soluble and insoluble. They are both important in the diet but perform different functions. How can you tell which fiber is soluble or insoluble? If you peel an apple and place the peel in a glass of water and stir it around, nothing happens (it doesn't dissolve in the water). This is an example of insoluble fiber. In general, bran and the skins and peels of fruits and vegetables contain insoluble fiber, which helps with constipation because it speeds the food through your gastrointestinal tract. If you take the pulp of an apple, on the other hand, and submerge it in water, you'll find it dissolves. This is an example of soluble fiber (e.g., applesauce). Soluble fiber may help with lowering cholesterol in some cases (e.g., oatmeal), and may also help if you're having diarrhea, because it is a natural stool binder.

The American Cancer Society recommends that 25 to 30 grams of fiber be included in our daily diet to potentially lower the risk for colon cancer, and possibly other cancers as well. Fiber also tends to help us feel fuller because it slows down the rate of blood sugar release and stomach emptying.

If you recently had weight-loss surgery, your center may recommend that you not include fiber in your diet during the first weeks or even months after your surgery to ensure that your new stomach and connection are working properly. Even if you did not have surgery that affects absorption (e.g., gastric banding), your surgical center may ask you not to include fiber in your diet for a while, especially after an adjustment or fill, since the narrowing from your pouch to the lower part of your stomach may be much more narrow, and too much fiber too soon may cause intolerance issues. As always, please check with your surgical center for specific dietary recommendations.

Vitamin and Minerals

Many surgical centers will do blood tests prior to your weight-loss surgery to ensure that you're in the best possible health before going into the operating room. It's not uncommon for people to have some vitamin and mineral deficiencies, so don't be alarmed if your doctor tells you that these deficiencies need to be corrected preceding surgery. I have found several studies citing Vitamin D deficiency or issues with iron, anemia, or Vitamin B12 before surgery.

It's important to take the prescription your doctor gives you to be in as good nutritional shape as possible before your life-changing weight-loss surgery. After surgery, it will be imperative to take your vitamins (with minerals) and calcium with Vitamin D, as well as any other supplements or medications prescribed for you.

If you are told that you have a vitamin or mineral deficiency after your surgery (and you've been taking all the supplements your doctor has ordered), don't be too hard on yourself. Studies show that even people who follow a healthy diet and take their recommended supplements following their surgery may have some deficiencies, so it might be that you need some additional supplementation. If not corrected right away, a Vitamin B12 deficiency may cause numbness or tingling in your fingers and memory loss. If not corrected for several weeks or months, it may even cause irreparable neurological damage. Thiamin, another B vitamin (vitamin B1, to be exact), is very dangerous if it gets low, since the plummet can happen very rapidly, and, in rare cases, can result in death! Please keep in mind this is highly uncommon, but if you have chronic vomiting and/or have new onset of burning and/or numbness in your feet, contact your center immediately since complications due to a thiamin deficiency can progress very quickly, and you certainly want to catch it before it results in something serious. My patients who have reported new onset of burning in their feet have told me that within one day they weren't able to feel their ankles. After IV thiamin treatment, they were almost as good as new the next day. Catching it quickly is key!

Don't be alarmed, dear readers. These deficiencies are fairly rare, especially if you follow your center's recommended course of dietary supplementation, eat right, and have your blood tests done at time points advised by your surgical center. Remember, the vitamin/mineral regimen is for a lifetime, not just for the immediate weeks or months after surgery. If you don't like the vitamin you're taking, talk to your surgical team, including your dietitian, to find an alternative. Keep in mind that solid vitamins/minerals and calcium may get stuck or may not be as well absorbed as chewable, liquid, or powder varieties. Time-released or enteric coated vitamins, supplements, and medications also may be poorly absorbed, especially after a procedure like gastric bypass surgery. So, the benefits of repairing your deficiencies are well worth it.

ARTIFICIAL SWEETENERS: HOW SWEET THEY ARE

Artificial sweeteners, also known as sugar substitutes, are designed to replace table sugar (or sucrose) in order to sweeten foods and beverages. You need to use less sugar substitute than sugar because artificial sweeteners are many times sweeter than table sugar. These sweeteners are regulated by the U.S. Food and Drug Administration (FDA).

Here are the most common artificial sweeteners found on the market and some general information regarding their uses:

SPLENDA (SUCRALOSE)

This artificial sweetener was approved by the FDA as a tabletop sweetener in 1998, and then as a general-purpose sweetener in 1999. Splenda is often regarded as "natural" because it's made from real sugar, although it's chemically combined with chlorine, a process most would consider unnatural. Splenda is 600 times sweeter than table sugar. It may be of benefit for people with diabetes, because it has been deemed to have no effect on carbohydrate metabolism, short- or long-term blood sugar control, or insulin secretion.

Splenda is considered to be very stable, so it's a popular ingredient in almost every type of food and beverage, including diet sodas, juice drinks, and teas. However, the biggest selling point is the ability to bake with Splenda, which isn't possible with most of the other artificial sweeteners.

EQUAL AND NUTRASWEET (ASPARTAME)

Aspartame, distributed under the trade names Equal and Nutrasweet, was approved in 1981 by the FDA, and it became the artificial sweetener of choice when saccharin decreased in popularity many years ago. It's derived from the amino acids (building blocks of protein) aspartic acid and phenylalanine. People who have a rare genetic disorder called PKU (phenylketonuria) can't break down phenylalanine, so they must totally avoid aspartame. However, it has been deemed safe for people with diabetes, as it seems to produce a very small rise in blood sugar.

This sweetener is 200 times sweeter than table sugar, and it is often used in beverages, ice cream, and puddings. Aspartame's sweetness is enhanced by other flavors and sweeteners, but it loses its sweetness when heated. Therefore, it is not ideal for baking. However, Sugar Lite, a new product that is a combination of table sugar and aspartame, can be used in baking. One teaspoon of this product contains 8 calories, which is half the calories of a teaspoon of pure table sugar.

SWEET'N LOW AND SUGAR TWIN (SACCHARIN)

Saccharin, which is sold as Sweet'N Low and Sugar Twin, is the oldest of the approved artificial sweeteners. In 1977, the FDA tried to ban saccharin based on research indicating it caused cancer in animals. However, it remained on the shelves, but with a warning regarding this finding. In 2000, the National Institutes of Health (NIH) removed saccharin from its list of cancer-causing agents (carcinogens), and the necessity of including the warning label regarding the animal studies was waived. Although saccharin has been cleared by the FDA, it continues to be a bit controversial.

Like other artificial sweeteners, saccharine produces no sugar (or glycemic) response. It is 300 times sweeter than table sugar, and it is used in many products. Sugar Twin, which is a combination of maltodextrin and sodium saccharin, contains 0 calories per teaspoon, but it measures the same as sugar, cup for cup. However, the label on the box states that Sugar Twin is not appropriate for recipes calling for more than ½ cup of sugar. Therefore, this product is not ideal for baking overall. It may be ideal though, for sweetening coffee or tea.

STEVIA (SWEET LEAF)

This sweetener is considered the ultimate "natural" sweetener, and it has been quite popular lately in the United States. It is extracted from a shrub that grows in South America. Because our bodies can't metabolize sweet leaf or break it down, it does not provide calories.

SUNETTE (ACESULFAME POTASSIUM)

This artificial sweetener was approved by the FDA in 1988. It is 200 times sweeter than table sugar, and it produces no blood sugar response. It is often found in diet sodas, juice drinks, gums, and ice cream. However, it's not available for use in baking or cooking.

SUGAR ALCOHOLS (SORBITOL, MANNITOL)

For many years, people with diabetes have used products with sugar alcohols—such as sorbitol, mannitol, xylitol, and maltitol—to sweeten foods without the sugar or glycemic response seen with table sugar. These are natural sweeteners that do not trigger an insulin reaction. Sugar alcohols contain half the calories of sugar, and they are not digested by the small intestine.

It is important to realize that sorbitol, one of the sugar alcohols commonly found on the market, is a natural laxative, and it may cause diarrhea, bloating, and flatulence. I often tell my patients not to try sugar alcohols for the first time while you're on a camping trip, since the potential laxative effect could be quite embarrassing and uncomfortable. However, for people having constipation issues, sugar-alcohol-sweetened products, in moderation, may help alleviate this problem. It is often found in sugar-free candies, as well as some high-protein bars.

Try these websites for more information regarding artificial sweeteners:

Splenda: www.splenda.com

Sweet'N Low: www.sweetnlow.com

Equal: www.equal.com

Sugar Twin: www.sugartwin.com

Saccharin: www.saccharin.org

PROTEIN POWDERS: WHAT'S THE SCOOP?

In this section, we discuss commonly found, high-quality protein powders, starting with the most commonly found and recommended variety, whey protein powder. It's important to check with your medical center's dietitian regarding the protein quality score (Protein Digestibility-Corrected Amino Score, or PDCAAS), which relates to the quality and absorption of the protein powders. I always discourage poor-quality protein, such as collagen (often marketed as "test tubes," "bullets," or "shots"); it's not highly absorbed, even if it's fortified, due to missing amino acids, or building blocks of protein, that our bodies cannot make. Some studies suggest absorption to be anywhere from 15 to 40 percent of the protein those collagen-based and/or "predigested" protein supplements claim you're getting. There are also a number of newer vegetarian protein powder options, including hemp, but their protein absorption may be suboptimal. In general, it's better to stick with whey or soy protein isolate, since they're lactose free and well digested and absorbed. Many of my weight-loss surgery patients ask me about protein powders, and it seems there are new ones cropping up almost daily. How do you know which ones are best? Also, are there any possible things to watch out for with some of the protein powders, such as intolerance issues?

Protein powders can vary greatly in terms of quality, and they may be a mixture of two or more different kinds of proteins. In terms of pure sources of protein, there are four general types: whey, soy, egg, and rice. Let's talk about each in turn.

WHEY PROTEIN

This is taken from milk, and is the most popular type of protein supplement on the market. Because it is a derivative of milk, it contains some lactose, or milk sugar. People who are lactose intolerant shouldn't take whey protein. Also, because gastric bypass and biliopancreatic diversion patients may have lactose intolerance issues after surgery, whey protein can cause a problem. If you have gas, abdominal bloating, cramping, and/or diarrhea every time you take whey protein, you may be lactose intolerant. Try taking the whey protein along with the enzyme lactase, which you can purchase over the counter at any pharmacy and many supermarkets. When taken with whey protein powder, this enzyme should eliminate the problem by breaking down the milk sugar (lactose) to lactic acid, thereby doing away with the symptoms.

Whey protein powders contain both essential amino acids (building blocks of protein the body cannot make) and nonessential amino acids (building blocks of protein that can be made in the body). Whey is easily taken up and used by the muscles in the body, and it is considered very safe to use.

There are two types of whey protein powders: concentrate and isolate. The concentrate form is more common, easier to find, and less expensive. It contains between 30 and 85 percent protein. Whey isolate is a higher quality protein, so it's more expensive than the concentrate. Because whey isolate contains more than 90 percent protein, it's more easily absorbed by the body, and it also contains less fat and lactose (milk sugar).

Benefits of whey protein: Whey protein may help boost immunity. It is an ideal source of amino acids. It also may help prevent muscle breakdown and speed up muscle recovery after exercise.

SOY PROTEIN

Soy protein comes from soy flour, so it is a good protein source for vegans. Soy is the most complete vegetable protein available. Like whey protein powders, soy protein also has two varieties: concentrate and isolate. The isolate is the more expensive form, because it is more pure and has a higher percentage of protein, compared to the concentrate. Soy protein is typically very easy to digest, and it can be considered as high a quality protein as milk and meat. I often recommend soy protein powders to my weight-loss surgery patients who have a milk allergy or lactose intolerance issues.

Benefits of soy protein: Soy protein is ideal for vegans, and it's perfect for people with milk intolerance or allergies. There are studies suggesting moderate soy consumption may help lower cholesterol and possibly reduce the risk of heart disease, although some recent studies seem to be challenging this claim.

EGG PROTEIN

Egg protein powders are made from egg whites, so they are very high in protein and essentially fat-free. Egg protein is considered a perfect protein, with a grade of 100 in terms of biological value. Egg protein is complete in essential amino acids, and it also has other amino acids, such as branched chain amino acids (leucine, isoleucine, and valine) and glutamic acid. The branched chain amino acids and glutamic acid may be especially useful after weight-loss surgery, because they tend to help muscles recover more quickly. However, egg protein powders should not be used by anyone with an egg allergy.

Benefits of egg protein: Egg protein is fat-free, fairly inexpensive, and not an issue for people with milk or lactose intolerance or soy intolerance or sensitivity.

RICE PROTEIN

Rice protein is made by carefully extracting the protein from brown rice. Although rice is often overlooked because of its incomplete amino acids, or building blocks of protein, rice powders are typically supplemented with L-amino acids to make them complete.

Benefits of rice protein: Rice protein is hypoallergenic, so it's ideal for people with soy, milk, or egg allergies or sensitivities. It is also perfect for vegans or strict vegetarians.

LYNETTE'S TIPS FOR STOCKING AN EFFICIENT KITCHEN

I can't count the number of times I've heard people say, "If only I could just make a few things turn out right in the kitchen!" Maybe you've uttered the same words. We are so pleased to present this cookbook to you that will guide you step-by-step through producing these user-friendly and delicious recipes and also help you become aware of some basic and essential culinary rules to live by. From cooking for your family to entertaining, there is something here for everyone. Let's begin with your kitchen. Here are a few good tips to follow to make your culinary adventures easy, fun, and educational.

It's essential to have a few standard pieces of equipment in your kitchen, which will make preparing any meal faster. A set of good sharp knives is an absolute must, along with a block to store them in to keep them from becoming dull quickly. A chef's blade (8- to 10-inch, or 20 to 25 cm), a fillet or boning knife, a serrated knife, and a small paring knife will get you through just about any recipe you'll ever prepare.

A pair of ordinary kitchen shears is also a good idea. Shears are wonderful for removing skin and fat from meat and poultry, for trimming vegetables of their stems and other unwanted parts, and for opening stubborn packages.

A set of nonstick pots and pans is a good item to have. Choose one that has thicker-gauged bottoms, which will promote even heat distribution and help to avoid constant scorching. Find the set that looks right for you in your local department store. A 7- or 9-piece set is sufficient to begin with, and then as you become more adventurous, you'll soon learn what additional pieces you wish to add to your collection.

Next, **a set of stainless-steel mixing bowls** can make your kitchen endeavors easier and more efficient. I prefer stainless steel over glass or plastic because it is light-weight but sturdy enough to handle an electric mixer or being dropped without breaking. In addition to being sturdy, stainless steel holds temperatures more efficiently than plastic or glass, neither of which conducts heat or cold. In other words, the item you are mixing in stainless steel will hold its temperature longer rather than rise or fall to room temperature like it will in glass or plastic. Choose a set of mixing bowls ranging in size from 1 to 5 quarts (1 to 5 liters) to meet all of your mixing needs. When mixing anything in your mixing bowls, be sure to leave plenty of room for the product to be sufficiently manipulated. Always use a bowl that is twice the size of the product you are mixing.

A food processor is essential for preparing purees and certain types of sauces. A blender can be used in place of a food processor. However, a blender may not be sufficient for certain applications, such as finely chopping onions and peppers or grinding meat and other products. Since blenders are essentially designed for liquids, gravity plays an important role in their design. A food processor, however, is designed to expose more surface area of the product being processed by the working blade and so that gravity is not such a factor. There are a variety of processors on the market today, and you can buy a decent one at a department store.

It is a good idea to keep **one colander** and **one fine mesh strainer or sieve** in your kitchen. It is important to wash vegetables before preparing them, and these are the tools to use. You will find many other uses for these simple and inexpensive items as well.

Eventually you will learn what works best for your kitchen and your own style as it develops. That's true for kitchen equipment, but also for food. Here are a few of my own essentials items I recommend having on hand at all times.

Ordinary table salt may be easily accessible, although it may not be the best choice for cooking. A **good sea salt** can be found at the grocer, as well as **kosher salt.** A little bit of either of these salts goes a long way.

Fresh cracked or fresh ground pepper can have a great deal more flavor compared to prepackaged ground pepper. Oil in the peppercorn dehydrates at a much faster rate after it is ground, and so the flavor dissipates as well. Truly fresh black pepper will have a fruity aroma and a hearty bite. In addition, I find that it's worth researching where your spices come from. Dried spices and seasonings will lose the intensity of flavor as they age. Quality ingredients, including spices and seasonings, can contribute a world of difference to your recipes.

Lemons are also essential in your kitchen. You will find many recipes in this book that require fresh lemon juice and lemon zest. Zest is the outer portion of the rind that is grated off with a zester or a fine grating surface. The flavor is very intense, and not at all bitter like the inner white portion of the rind. You will also find recipes using fresh lime and orange zest.

There are many **substitutes available for butter,** such as light butters, margarines, and butter alternatives. I recommend reduced-fat and reduced-calorie butter in place of margarine, because of the usually high sodium content in margarine. Some spreads contain olive oil and offer a rich flavor and good heat conduction when using for a sauté. When using a butter alternative or oil to sauté foods, always be sure to thoroughly heat it before adding the ingredients to be sautéed, unless the recipe states otherwise.

Quite a few recipes in the book call for **wine.** If you prefer not to cook using alcohol, any of our recipes calling for the use of wine can be made without compromising flavor or consistency simply by substituting chicken or vegetable broth or water with a bit of lemon juice for the wine.

You'll find that the recipes often offer ranges of time for cooking, such as bake for 20 to 30 minutes, instead of exact numbers. That's because each oven, stovetop, refrigerator, and freezer varies in temperature. Likewise, different pots, pans, and baking dishes will all conduct temperatures to varying degrees, and so it is necessary to make adjustments to cooking time and temperatures as you progress through any recipe.

As you're cooking, to save time and also to stay organized in your kitchen, it's always best to have all of the measured, cut, and prepared ingredients ready to use before you begin the recipe.

Here's an important food safety note. **It's important to keep the work surfaces, such as counter tops and cutting boards, clean and sanitized.** An ordinary kitchen sponge will transfer concentrated amounts of bacteria from every surface it has touched since it was placed into use. One of the best solutions for sanitizing is simply bleach and tap water, in the proportion of one capful of bleach to one gallon of water. If too much bleach is used, the solution will evaporate before it has sufficient time to sanitize. Also, bleach in the solution will evaporate if the temperature of the water is too hot.

Now that you have the basic recommendations for setting up your kitchen, we hope all of your culinary endeavors are delicious, nutritious, exciting, and fun!

CHAPTER 1

Breakfasts and Brunches

All-American Scramble

TEXTURE: SOFT

To save time, prepare the turkey bacon ahead of time per the package instructions. Serve this, or any of the scrambles in this book, with a slice of whole grain toast or English muffin for a complete breakfast. You can leave out the cheese from any of these scrambles.

1 teaspoon light butter

1 slice turkey bacon, crumbled

¼ cup (60 ml) liquid egg substitute

1 tablespoon (7 g) reduced-fat shredded Cheddar cheese

—

Yield: Makes 1 serving

In an omelet pan, melt the butter over medium heat, swirling the pan to coat evenly.

Add the turkey bacon and sauté 4 to 5 minutes, until it becomes soft and just begins to brown. Add the egg substitute, stirring gently but constantly with a heat-resistant rubber spatula, scraping the bottom of the pan to keep the eggs moving to avoid browning. When the eggs are almost finished, add the cheese and turn off the heat. Gently fold the cheese into the eggs, turning over with the spatula. When the cheese becomes soft, but not dissolved, turn the scramble onto a plate.

NUTRITIONAL ANALYSIS

EACH WITH: Calories: 118.13, Protein: 11.03 g, Carbs: 0.59 g, Total Fat: 7.89 g, Sat Fat: 2.09 g, Cholesterol: 14.38 mg, Sodium: 379.82 mg, Sugars: 0.40 g, Fiber: 0.00 g

Mushroom and Swiss Cheese Scramble

TEXTURE: SOFT

1 teaspoon light butter

¼ cup (15 g) sliced mushrooms

¼ cup (60 ml) liquid egg substitute

1 slice (1 ounce, or 28 g) low-fat Swiss cheese, cut into strips

—

Yield: Makes 1 serving

In an omelet pan over medium heat, melt the butter, swirling the pan to coat evenly.

Add the mushrooms and sauté about 4 to 5 minutes, until they become soft and just begin to brown. Add the egg substitute, stirring gently but constantly with a heat-resistant rubber spatula, scraping the bottom of the pan to keep the eggs moving to avoid browning. When the eggs are almost finished, add the cheese and turn off the heat. Gently fold the cheese into the eggs, turning over with the rubber spatula. When the cheese becomes soft but not dissolved, turn the scramble onto a plate.

NUTRITIONAL ANALYSIS

EACH WITH: Calories: 171.85, Protein: 19.29 g, Carbs: 2.24 g, Total Fat: 9.27 g, Sat Fat: 3.57 g, Cholesterol: 17.63 mg, Sodium: 223.34 mg, Sugars: 1.46 g, Fiber: 0.68 g

Greek Scramble

TEXTURE: SOFT

1 teaspoon light butter

½ teaspoon chopped fresh thyme leaves

¼ cup (60 ml) liquid egg substitute

2 large pitted black olives, sliced

2 teaspoons finely diced green bell pepper

2 teaspoons feta cheese crumbles

—

Yield: Makes 1 serving

In an omelet pan over medium heat, melt the butter, swirling the pan to coat evenly. Add the thyme and sauté about 1 to 2 minutes, until it begins to bubble and sweat. Add the egg substitute, stirring gently but constantly with a heat-resistant rubber spatula, scraping the bottom of the pan to keep the eggs moving to avoid browning. When the eggs are almost finished, add the olives, pepper, and cheese and turn off the heat. Gently fold the ingredients into the eggs, turning over with the rubber spatula. When the cheese becomes soft but not dissolved, turn the scramble onto a plate.

NUTRITIONAL ANALYSIS

EACH WITH: Calories: 96.95, Protein: 8.61 g, Carbs: 1.78 g, Total Fat: 5.97 g, Sat Fat: 1.68 g, Cholesterol: 6.19 mg, Sodium: 247.13 mg, Sugars: 1.42 g, Fiber: 0.38 g

Fresh Herb and Goat Cheese Scramble

1 teaspoon light butter
1 teaspoon chopped fresh parsley
1 teaspoon chopped fresh chives
1 teaspoon chopped fresh tarragon
¼ cup (60 ml) liquid egg substitute
2 teaspoons goat cheese crumbles

—

Yield: Makes 1 serving

In an omelet pan over medium heat, melt the butter, swirling the pan to coat evenly.

Add the parsley, chives, and tarragon and sauté 1 to 2 minutes, until they begin to bubble and sweat. Add the egg substitute, stirring gently but constantly with a heat-resistant rubber spatula, scraping the bottom of the pan to keep the eggs moving to avoid browning. When the eggs are almost finished, add the cheese and turn off the heat. Gently fold the cheese into the eggs, turning over with the spatula. When the cheese becomes soft but not dissolved, turn the scramble onto a plate.

NUTRITIONAL ANALYSIS

EACH WITH: Calories: 103.94, Protein: 9.90 g, Carbs: 0.98 g, Total Fat: 6.66 g, Sat Fat: 2.51 g, Cholesterol: 8.07 mg, Sodium: 166.70 mg, Sugars: 0.58 g, Fiber: 0.11 g

Italian Scramble

TEXTURE: SOFT

1 teaspoon light butter
⅛ teaspoon dried oregano
2 teaspoons finely chopped yellow onion
1 tablespoon (10 g) chopped tomato
¼ cup (60 ml) liquid egg substitute
1 slice (1 ounce, or 28 g) part skim mozzarella, cut into strips

—

Yield: Makes 1 serving

In an omelet pan over medium heat, melt the butter, swirling the pan to coat evenly. Add the oregano and sauté 4 to 5 minutes, until it begins to sweat. Add the onions and continue cooking, until they become soft. Add the tomato and stir just enough to evenly distribute. Add the egg substitute, stirring gently but constantly with a heat-resistant rubber spatula, scraping the bottom of the pan to keep the eggs moving to avoid browning. When the eggs are almost finished, add the cheese and turn off the heat. Gently fold the cheese into the eggs, turning over with the spatula. When the cheese becomes soft but not dissolved, turn the scramble onto a plate.

NUTRITIONAL ANALYSIS

EACH WITH: Calories: 158.21, Protein: 15.05 g, Carbs: 1.86 g, Total Fat: 9.63 g, Sat Fat: 4.41 g, Cholesterol: 18.92 mg, Sodium: 343.86 mg, Sugars: 1.08 g, Fiber: 0.27 g

Spanish Omelet

This is a delicious (and nutritious) way to start your day!

3 teaspoons drained and chopped roasted red pepper

2 tablespoons (20 g) chopped tomato

½ teaspoon fresh minced garlic

3 or four 1-inch (2.5-cm) button mushrooms, cleaned and sliced

2 tablespoons (20 g) 95% fat-free ham, diced

¼ cup (60 ml) liquid egg substitute

1 slice soy cheese, cut into strips

1½ teaspoons fresh cilantro, chopped

2 tablespoons (35 g) Fresh Salsa Caliente (page 82)

Fresh strawberries

—

Yield: Makes 2 (about ½-cup) servings

Coat a 6-inch (15-cm) nonstick omelet pan with cooking spray and heat to medium high.

Add the roasted pepper, tomato, garlic, mushrooms, and ham and sauté for about 4 minutes, or until the mushrooms are soft. Transfer the mixture to a bowl, drain off excess liquid, and set aside.

Wipe clean the pan with paper towels and coat again with nonstick spray. Heat over medium heat and add the egg substitute. Using a rubber spatula, carefully lift the sides of the omelet up to let the egg substitute spill underneath the cooked, solid bottom. Repeat this process until the egg mixture is almost done, then turn off the heat. Immediately add the cheese and cilantro to the bottom half of the omelet, followed by the sauté mixture. Gently fold the top half of the omelet over the bottom half and carefully slide it onto a serving plate. Top the omelet with the salsa and garnish the plate with the strawberries.

NUTRITIONAL ANALYSIS

EACH WITH: Calories: 83.85, Protein: 10.21 g, Carbs: 5.15 g, Total Fat: 3.77 g, Sat Fat: 0.52 g, Cholesterol: 7.12 mg, Sodium: 303.63 mg, Sugars: 3.13 g, Fiber: 0.84 g

Mark's Fruity French Toast

Mark is a gastric bypass surgery patient in the Boston area who makes this recipe for himself almost every morning and loves it.

¼ cup (60 ml) liquid egg substitute

1 tablespoon (14 ml) nonfat milk

½ teaspoon allspice

2 slices reduced-calorie whole-wheat bread

¼ cup (40 g) sliced fresh strawberries

⅓ cup (50 g) fresh blueberries

⅛ cup (30 ml) sugar-free maple syrup

—

Yield: Makes 1 (2-slice) serving

Coat a medium (big enough to hold two slices of bread) nonstick pan with cooking spray.

In a small mixing bowl combine the egg substitute, milk, and allspice. Dip the bread into the egg batter to coat both sides.

Heat the pan over medium heat. Place the bread into the pan and cook on both sides, until golden brown. Transfer the French toast to a serving plate and top with the strawberries, blueberries, and maple syrup.

NUTRITIONAL ANALYSIS

EACH WITH: Calories: 221.36, Protein: 12.91 g, Carbs: 39.31 g, Total Fat: 3.52 g, Sat Fat: 0.63 g, Cholesterol: 0.93 mg, Sodium: 408.18 mg, Sugars: 9.14 g, Fiber: 7.65 g

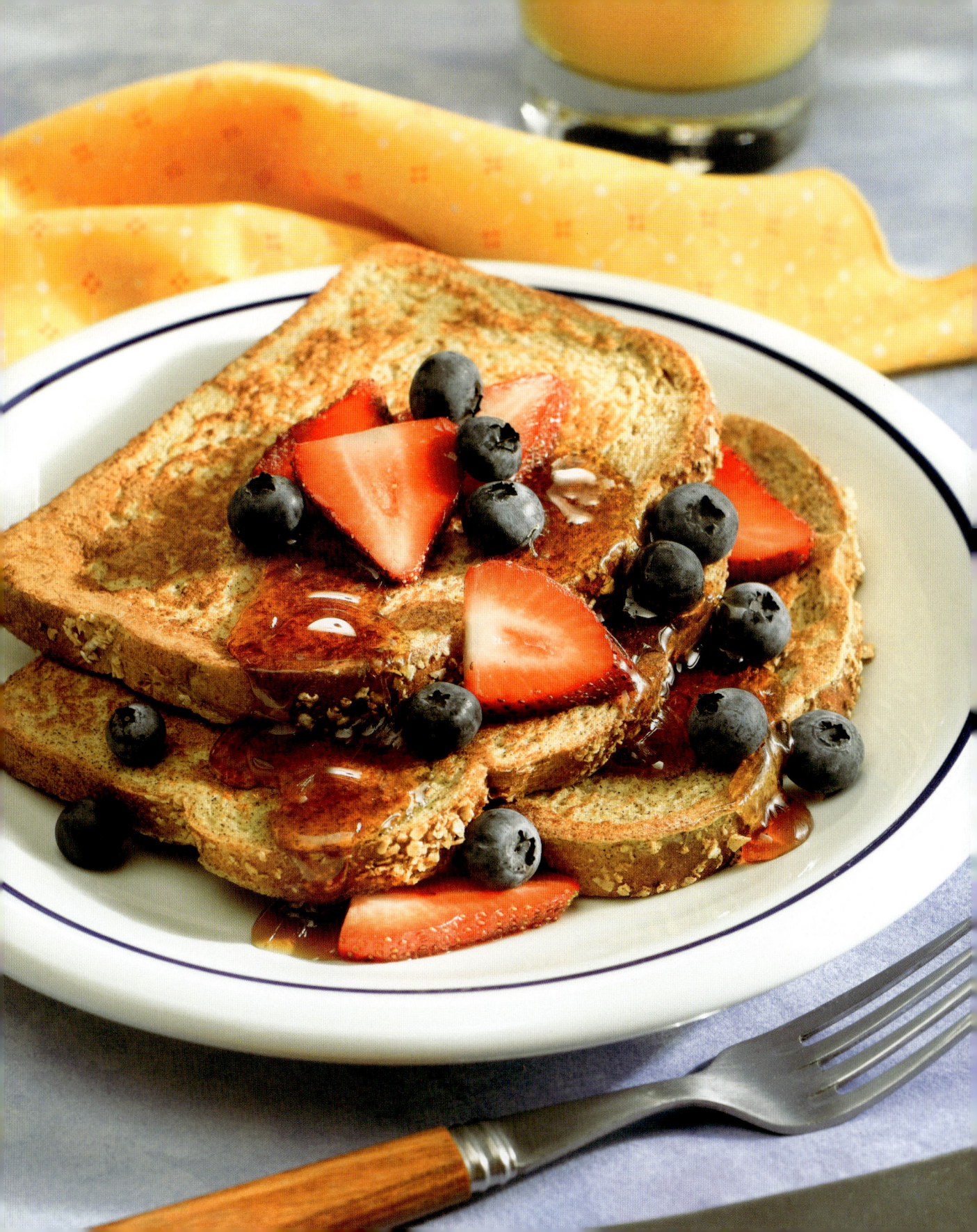

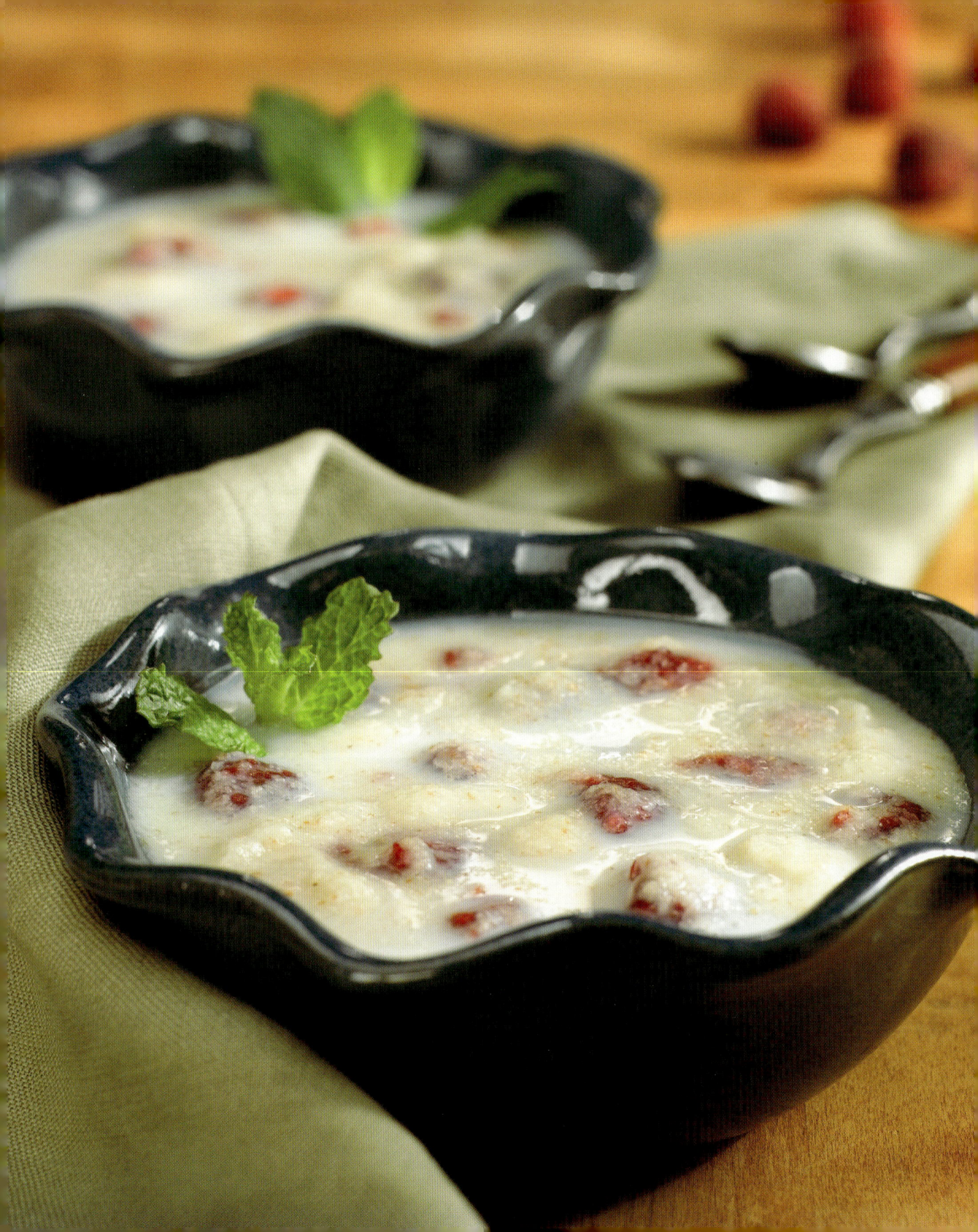

Berry Delicious Cream of Wheat

TEXTURE: SOFT

"Very satisfying and filling."

—Julie, *a gastric bypass surgery patient in the Boston area*

¾ cup (135 g) instant Cream of Wheat, no salt added

½ teaspoon vanilla extract

½ cup (60 g) fresh raspberries

2 tablespoons (15 g) protein powder supplement (see note)

2 tablespoons (28 ml) nonfat milk or low-fat, low-sugar soy milk

2 sprigs spearmint

—

Yield: Makes 2 servings

Prepare Cream of Wheat per the package instruction for 2 servings, adding the vanilla to the water before boiling. Just before removing the Cream of Wheat from the pan, stir in the raspberries. Add the protein powder just prior to serving. Serve in warmed bowls, topped with the milk and garnished with fresh spearmint sprigs.

NUTRITIONAL ANALYSIS

EACH WITH: Calories: 219.29, Protein: 24.88 g, Carbs: 23.10 g, Total Fat: 3.21 g, Sat Fat: 0.07 g, Cholesterol: 0.28 mg, Sodium: 83.74 mg, Sugars: 4.04, Fiber: 4.36 g

MARGARET'S NOTES

• Although raspberries contain the highest fiber of all berries, you may substitute blueberries, blackberries, strawberries, or huckleberries.

• It is essential to select a protein powder that is appropriate for hot foods and beverages for this recipe to optimize the quality of the protein (avoid protein breakdown) when exposed to heat, a process known as denaturing. This is also why you add the protein powder after heating the Cream of Wheat, just prior to serving it.

Cumin Mushroom Omelet

This is simple and delicious! For a complete breakfast, serve this delicious omelet with a whole-wheat English muffin half and fresh fruit. Serve it with Fresh Salsa Caliente (page 82).

Serve it with Fresh Salsa Caliente (page 82).

TEXTURE: SOFT

½ pound (225 g) mushrooms

1 tablespoon (14 g) low-fat butter alternative

1 teaspoon olive oil

1 small clove garlic, minced

2 teaspoons ground cumin

⅛ teaspoon cayenne pepper (optional)

¼ teaspoon paprika

¼ teaspoon kosher salt or sea salt

2 tablespoons (25 g) nonfat sour cream

1 cup (235 ml) liquid egg substitute

¾ cup (85 g) reduced-fat shredded Cheddar cheese

¼ cup (4 g) chopped fresh cilantro

Fresh cilantro sprigs

—

Yield: Makes 4 (about ½-cup) servings

Clean the mushrooms with a mushroom brush or paper towels. Cut the end of the stems away and discard. Slice the mushrooms into thin slices.

In a medium nonstick skillet, heat the butter alternative and oil over medium heat. Add the mushrooms, garlic, cumin, pepper, paprika, and salt. Sauté, stirring often, for about 8 minutes, until the mushrooms become soft. Stir in the sour cream and continue cooking for 2 minutes, stirring once or twice. Remove the pan from the heat.

Coat a 7-inch (17.5 cm) nonstick skillet with cooking spray and heat to medium. Add the egg substitute and cook until the bottom becomes solid, but not browned. Using a rubber spatula, carefully lift the sides of the omelet up to let the egg substitute spill underneath the cooked, solid bottom. Repeat this process until the egg mixture is entirely cooked, then turn off the heat. Add the cheese and cilantro to the bottom half of the omelet. Fold the top half over the bottom half and gently press down with the rubber spatula. Cut the omelet in half and slide the halves onto serving plates. Garnish with the cilantro sprigs and salsa.

NUTRITIONAL ANALYSIS

EACH WITH: Calories: 160.93, Protein: 14.59 g, Carbs: 5.09 g, Total Fat: 9.11 g, Sat Fat: 3.39 g, Cholesterol: 13.13 mg, Sodium: 408.90 mg, Sugars: 1.99 g, Fiber: 1.19 g

Lisi's "Berry Kool" Smoothie

TEXTURE: PUREED. MAY BE ALLOWED ON SOME FULL LIQUID MEALS. This is a great smoothie to run out the door with in the morning; the sweet and tart taste of delicious fresh berries with the addition of extra vitamins and minerals found in the greens will really amp up your day. It was created by Lisi Deswart, dietetic intern at the University of Maryland Eastern Shore, class of 2011.

½ cup (65 g) fresh raspberries

½ cup (75 g) fresh blackberries

½ cup (115 g) 2% Greek yogurt

½ cup (120 ml) skim milk

2 stalks kale, leaves removed and finely chopped

—

Yield: Makes 2 (8-ounce) smoothies

Add the raspberries, blackberries, yogurt, milk, and kale leaves to blender. Blend until smooth.

NUTRITIONAL ANALYSIS

EACH WITH: Calories: 94.65, Protein: 8.11 g, Carbs: 14.67 g, Total Fat: 1.47 g, Sat Fat: 0.80 g, Cholesterol: 4.97 mg, Sodium: 52.02 mg, Sugars: 6.94 g, Fiber: 2.14 g

JOE'S TIP

To cut cost, it's perfectly fine to use frozen berries instead of fresh. Frozen berries are always good to have on hand for many recipes. Try them in different combinations to spice up your favorite protein powder.

Frozen Fruit Smoothie

TEXTURE: PUREED. MAY BE ALLOWED ON SOME FULL LIQUID MEALS

Frozen fruit smoothies can become a high-protein, easy-to-digest meal when you're on the go, or in the earlier stages of your postoperative diet. You can incorporate them into your diet up to twice a day if you're very busy or if you find your weight is inching upward and you'd like to reverse the trend. If you freeze the bananas for a few hours before making this shake, it will be even thicker and more delicious.

"I love this smoothie. My 3-year-old son loves it too, and we call it 'fruit milk.' It makes a tasty treat that has some nice chunks in it. This is great if you have no time and really want something yummy."

—Julie, *a gastric bypass patient in the New Bedford, Massachusetts, area*

4 ounces (115 g) banana, sliced (approximately 8- to 8⅞-inches long)

1 cup (150 g) fresh or frozen blueberries (see note)

1 cup (235 ml) soy milk, unsweetened (see note), or 1 to 1½ cups (235 ml) nonfat milk

2 ounces (55 g) protein powder supplement (see note)

2 sprigs mint

—
Yield: Makes 2 servings

In a blender, combine the bananas, blueberries, soy milk, and protein powder. Blend for 10 to 15 seconds, until a smooth consistency is reached. Garnish with the mint.

NUTRITIONAL ANALYSIS

EACH WITH: Calories: 250.73, Protein: 27.09 g, Carbs: 26.33 g, Total Fat: 5.01 g, Sat Fat: 0.06 g, Cholesterol: 0.00 mg, Sodium: 85.00 mg, Sugars: 13.93 g, Fiber: 5.47 g

NOTES

• Make sure the soy milk contains no more than 14 grams of sugars per cup.

• Generic (low-sugar) protein powders are fine, but please ensure they're appropriate for cold beverages.

MARGARET'S NOTE

You may substitute raspberries, straw-berries, or blackberries for the blue-berries, because the calories and carbohydrates are equivalent. Raspberries are the highest in fiber among these fruits, but all contain healthy antioxidants, which are wonderful cancer-fighting agents.

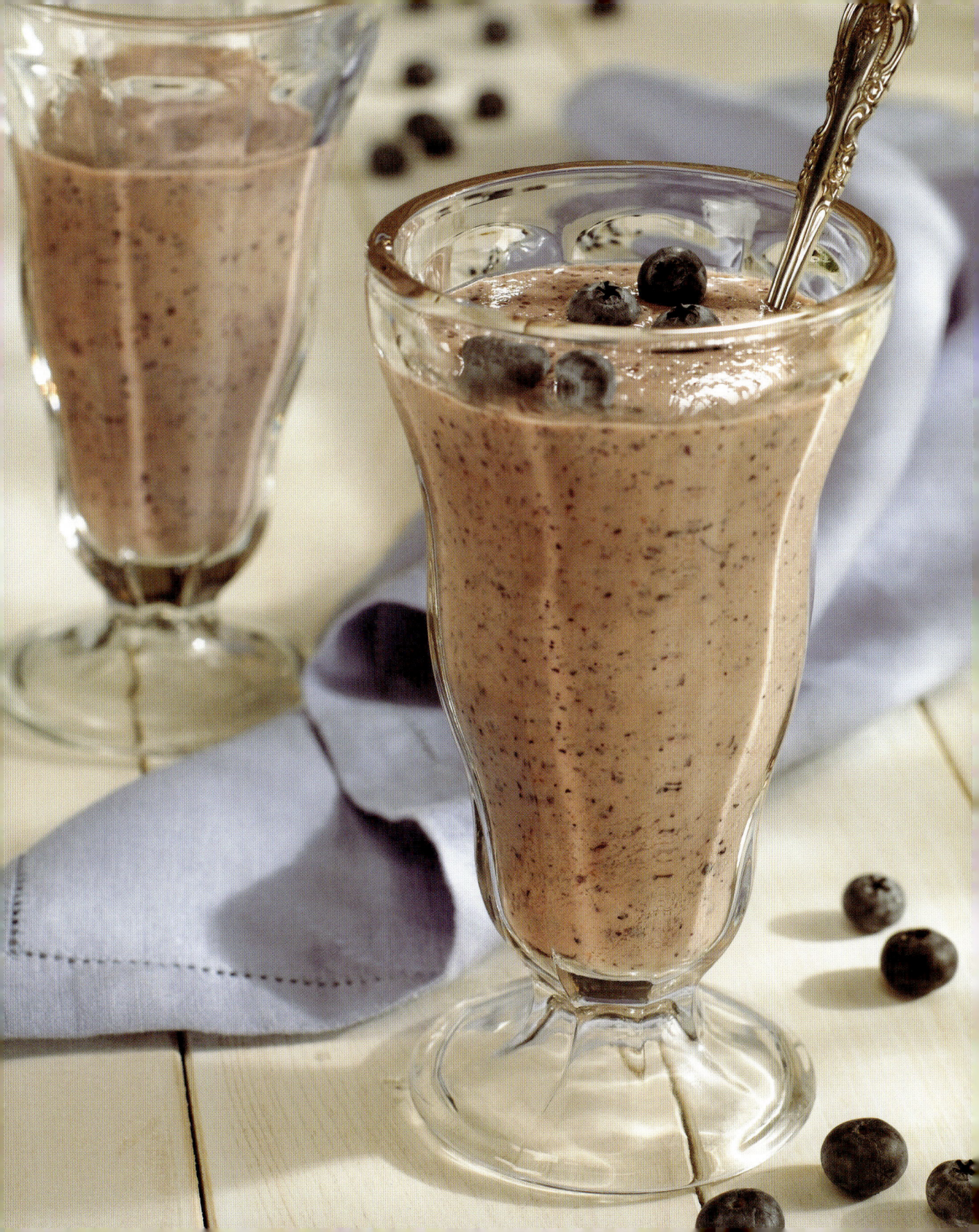

Zucchini Frittata with Capers and Olives

This is great served with the Chive-Yogurt Sauce on the next page.

2 teaspoons extra-virgin olive oil

2 cloves garlic, minced

½ cup (70 g) finely diced red bell pepper

1 cup (160 g) finely diced yellow onion

2 cups (250 g) grated zucchini

2 tablespoons (20 g) capers, drained

¼ cup (35 g) finely diced, pitted black or Greek olives

½ cup (75 g) feta cheese crumbles

2 tablespoons (8 g) chopped fresh parsley

2½ cups (590 ml) liquid egg substitute

—

Yield: Makes 6 (1½-cup) servings

Preheat the oven to 375°F (190°C, or gas mark 5). Spray cooking spray around the inside edges of an 8-inch (20-cm) cast iron skillet. In the skillet, heat the oil over medium-high, stirring occasionally. Sauté the garlic, bell pepper, and onion for about 5 minutes, until soft but not brown. Remove the skillet from heat and add the zucchini, capers, and olives. Arrange the cheese and parsley evenly over the sauté mixture. Slowly pour the egg substitute over the top of the mixture in the skillet.

Place the skillet in the oven and bake for 40 minutes, until the center of the frittata rises to match the outer edges. (The frittata should be just beginning to brown when it's finished cooking. If it begins to brown too quickly, reduce the oven temperature to 350°F, 180°C, or gas mark 4.) Serve on warmed plates with Chive-Yogurt Sauce drizzled over the top of each slice.

NUTRITIONAL ANALYSIS

EACH WITH: Calories: 172.69, Protein: 15.32 g, Carbs: 7.03 g, Total Fat: 8.86 g, Sat Fat: 2.80 g, Cholesterol: 12.17 mg, Sodium: 506.49 mg, Sugars: 4.01 g, Fiber: 1.25 g

Chive-Yogurt Sauce

TEXTURE: PUREED. MAY BE ALLOWED ON SOME FULL LIQUID MEALS.

This is a light, clean-tasting sauce that would be great with lamb, chicken, beef, and even as a dip for pita bread or vegetables.

¼ **cup (50 g) nonfat sour cream**

¼ **cup (60 g) nonfat plain yogurt**

½ **teaspoon salt**

⅛ **teaspoon ground white pepper**

1 **tablespoon finely chopped chives**

—

Yield: Makes 6 (1-tablespoon) servings

In a small mixing bowl, combine the sour cream, yogurt, salt, pepper, and chives. Vigorously mix with a fork or wire whip.

NUTRITIONAL ANALYSIS

EACH WITH: Calories: 16.13, Protein: 1.06 g, Carbs: 2.68 g, Total Fat: 0 g, Sat Fat: 0 g, Cholesterol: 1.88 mg, Sodium: 110.43 mg, Sugars: 1.30 g, Fiber: 0.03 g

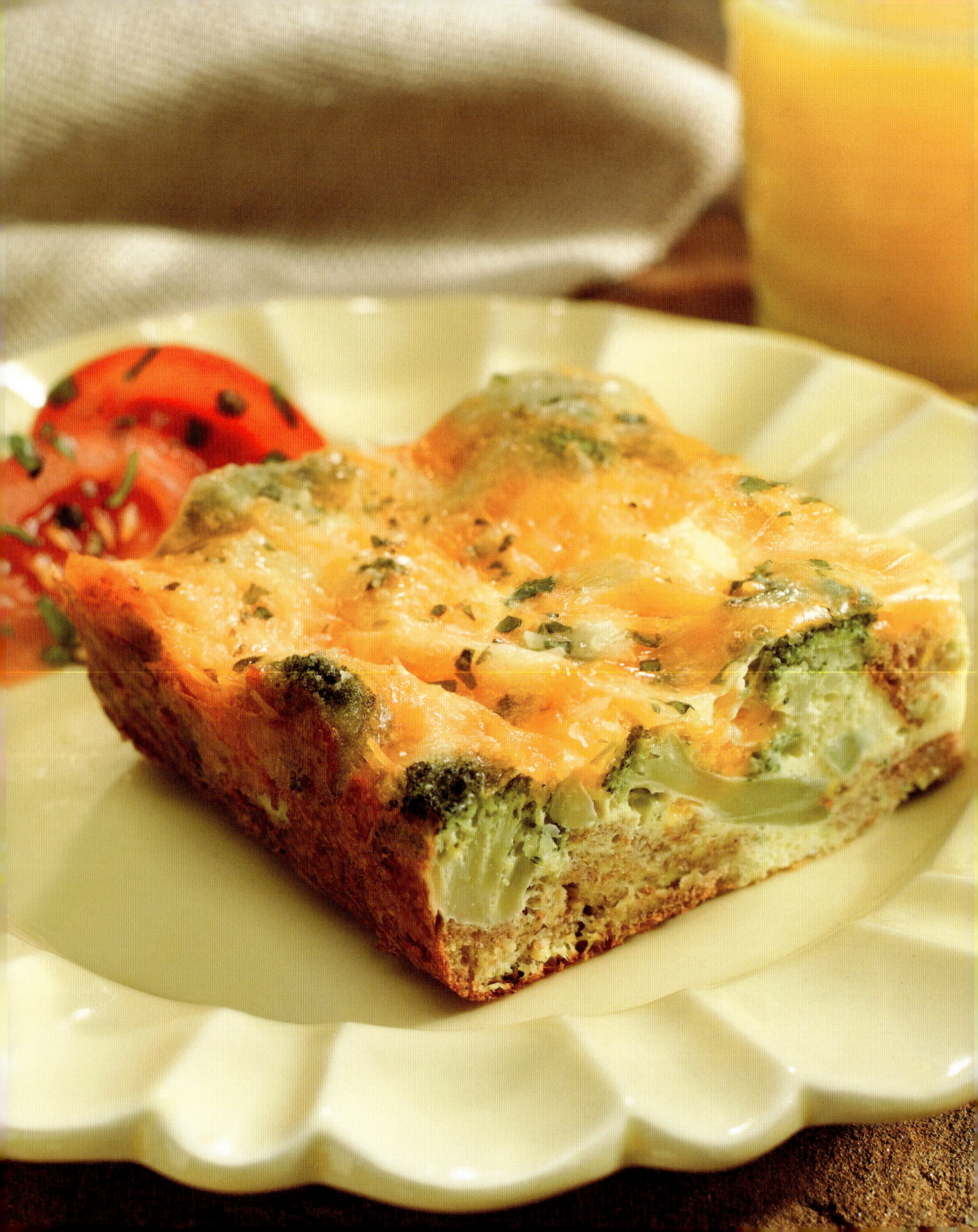

Savory Broccoli and Cheese Bread Pudding

TEXTURE: REGULAR

This is an elegant breakfast, lunch, or dinner.

2 teaspoons olive oil

1 medium sweet onion, diced (about 1½ cups, or 240 g)

½ teaspoon dried oregano

½ teaspoon dried basil

¼ teaspoon granulated garlic

5–6 whole-wheat English muffins, toasted and cut into ½-inch (1.25-cm) croutons

1 package (14 ounces, or 400 g) chopped frozen broccoli, thawed and drained

1½ cups (170 g) reduced-fat shredded Cheddar cheese

2 tablespoons (10 g) shredded Parmesan cheese

3 large eggs, beaten

2 tablespoons (8 g) chopped fresh parsley

½ cup (120 ml) nonfat half-and-half

—
Yield: Makes 12 (⅔-cup) servings

Preheat the oven to 350°F (180°C, or gas mark 4).

In a medium skillet, heat the oil over medium-high heat. Add the onion and sauté until it begins to soften. Add the oregano, basil, and garlic and continue cooking for an additional 2 minutes, stirring once or twice. Remove the mixture from heat and set aside.

Coat a 7- x 9-inch (17.5- x 22.5-cm) baking dish with cooking spray. Place the croutons and broccoli in the baking dish. Evenly distribute the sauté mixture over the bread and broccoli. Sprinkle the Cheddar and Parmesan over the croutons and broccoli.

In a small (1 quart, or 1 L) mixing bowl, combine the eggs, parsley, and half-and-half, then pour the egg mixture evenly over the cheese. Bake for 35 minutes, until the center of the dish has risen to meet the level at the edges and the top is golden brown.

NUTRITIONAL ANALYSIS

EACH WITH: Calories: 196.14, Protein: 11.01 g, Carbs: 25.80 g, Total Fat: 6.36 g, Sat Fat: 2.70 g, Cholesterol: 68.50 mg, Sodium: 480.27 mg, Sugars: 6.13 g, Fiber: 4.49 g

Breakfast Turkey Sausage Patties

TEXTURE: REGULAR

Serve these breakfast sausages with any of our egg dishes, frittatas, or egg scrambles and whole-wheat English muffins for a satisfying breakfast or brunch.

1 pound (455 g) lean ground turkey (93% fat-free or leaner)

¼ cup (25 g) fine, plain bread crumbs

2 teaspoons ground sage

1 teaspoon ground coriander

1 teaspoon ground oregano

½ teaspoon ground thyme

½ teaspoon black pepper

¼ teaspoon sea salt or kosher salt

¼ teaspoon cayenne pepper (optional)

½ teaspoon paprika

½ teaspoon garlic powder

½ cup (120 ml) low-sodium chicken broth

—

Yield: Makes 8 (about 2-ounce) patties

In a large (4 quart, or 4 L) mixing bowl, combine the turkey, bread crumbs, sage, coriander, oregano, thyme, black pepper, salt, cayenne pepper (if using), paprika, and garlic powder. Stir to incorporate completely. Add the broth, stir again, and let stand in the refrigerator for about 20 minutes. Form the mixture into 8 patties, about ½-inch (1.25 cm) thick.

Coat a nonstick skillet with cooking spray and heat over medium-high. Cook the patties for about 7 minutes on each side, until browned and done in the center.

NUTRITIONAL ANALYSIS

EACH WITH: Calories: 78.73, Protein: 14.25 g, Carbs: 3.32 g, Total Fat: 1.06 g, Sat Fat: 0.32 g, Cholesterol: 27.54 mg, Sodium: 166.32 mg, Sugars: 0.27 g, Fiber: 0.49 g

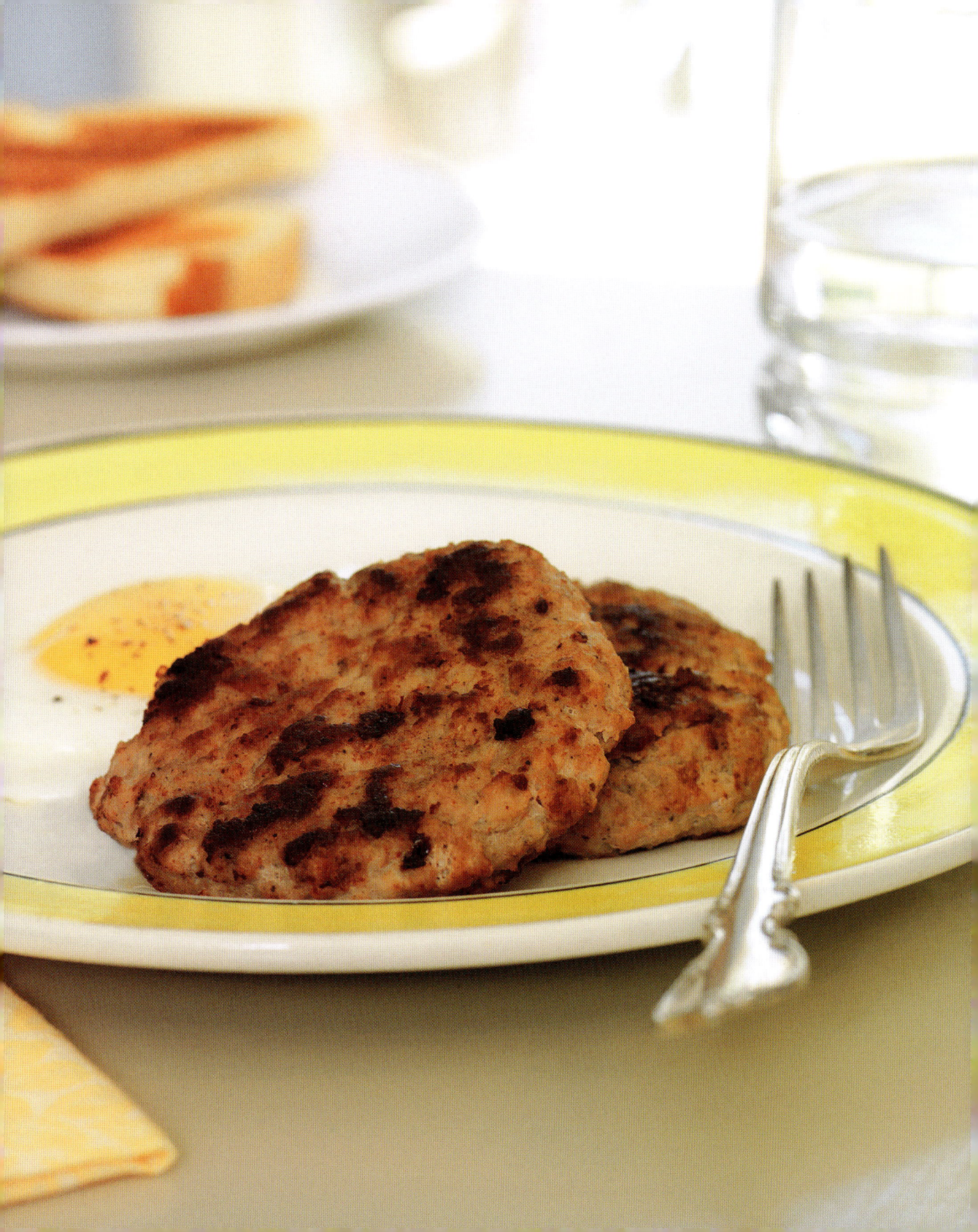

Carrot Muffins with Fresh Dill

TEXTURE: REGULAR

Serve these savory muffins with soup or salad for a special luncheon.

¼ cup (40 g) light brown sugar or brown sugar substitute (see note)

1 cup (110 g) oat bran flour

½ cup (55 g) all-purpose flour

1 teaspoon baking powder

1 teaspoon baking soda

1 teaspoon onion powder

½ teaspoon salt

1 egg

1 tablespoon (14 ml) vegetable oil

⅓ cup (65 g) sugar

1 teaspoon lemon juice

1 cup (240 g) nonfat plain or vanilla yogurt

¾ cup (85 g) finely grated carrots

2 tablespoons (4 g) chopped fresh dill

¼ cup (60 g) unsweetened applesauce

—

Yield: Makes 12 (about 2-ounce) muffins

Preheat the oven to 375°F (190°C, or gas mark 5). Spray a muffin tin with nonstick spray.

In a large mixing bowl, combine the light brown sugar, oat bran flour, all-purpose flour, baking powder, baking soda, onion powder, and salt. Stir to combine.

In a medium mixing bowl, whisk together the egg, oil, sugar, juice, yogurt, carrots, dill, and applesauce, just enough to combine. (The batter should be slightly lumpy.)

Fill the muffin cups two-thirds full with batter. Bake for 20 to 25 minutes, until a toothpick inserted into the middle of a muffin comes out clean. Let the muffins cool for 15 minutes before turning the tin over to release the muffins. (If the muffins stick to the pan, a slight tap on the back should help to release them.)

NUTRITIONAL ANALYSIS

EACH WITH: Calories: 104.71, Protein: 3.03 g, Carbs: 19.5 g, Total Fat: 2 g, Sat Fat: 0.22 g, Cholesterol: 20.42 mg, Sodium: 215.52 mg, Sugars: 6.63 g, Fiber: 1.59 g

MARGARET'S NOTE

If you leave out the brown sugar, each serving will provide: Calories: 90 Protein: 3 g Carbs: 15 g Total Fat: 2 g Sugars: 3 g. (The sugar substitute won't affect the saturated fat, cholesterol, sodium, or fiber.)

Fresh Strawberry Muffins

TEXTURE: REGULAR

When strawberries are in season, these muffins are as good for dessert as they are for breakfast.

⅓ cup (65 g) sugar or ⅓ cup (9 g) baking sugar substitute (see page 18) (see note)

1 cup (110 g) oat bran flour

½ cup (55 g) all-purpose flour

1 teaspoon baking powder

1 teaspoon baking soda

½ teaspoon salt

1 egg

1 tablespoon (14 ml) vegetable oil

1½ teaspoons vanilla extract

1 cup (240 g) nonfat vanilla yogurt

¼ cup (60 g) unsweetened applesauce

¾ cup (120 g) sliced fresh strawberries

—

Yield: Makes 12 (about 2-ounce) muffins

Preheat the oven to 375°F (190°C, or gas mark 5). Spray a muffin tin with nonstick spray.

In a large mixing bowl, combine the sugar or sugar substitute, oat bran flour, all-purpose flour, baking powder, baking soda, and salt. Stir to combine.

In a medium mixing bowl, whisk together the egg, oil, vanilla, yogurt, and applesauce, just enough to combine. (The batter should be slightly lumpy.) Gently fold in the strawberries.

Fill the muffin cups two-thirds full with batter. Bake for 20 to 25 minutes, until a toothpick inserted into the middle of a muffin comes out clean. Let the muffins cool for 15 minutes before turning the tin over to release the muffins. (If the muffins stick to the pan, a slight tap on the back should help to release them.)

NUTRITIONAL ANALYSIS

EACH WITH: Calories: 111.53, Protein: 2.94 g, Carbs: 21.11 g, Total Fat: 2 g, Sat Fat: 0.22 g, Cholesterol: 20.42 mg, Sodium: 205.71 mg, Sugars: 8.79 g, Fiber: 1.37 g

LYNETTE'S NOTE

For dessert: Slice a muffin in half horizontally and fill the middle with 2 tablespoons (35 g) nonfat, sugar-free vanilla pudding. Replace the top and add a dollop of nonfat whipped cream topping and a few fresh strawberry slices.

MARGARET'S NOTE

If you omit the sugar, each serving will provide: Calories: 88 Protein: 3 g Carbs: 15 g Total Fat: 2 g Sugars: 2 g. (The saturated fat, cholesterol, sodium, and fiber won't change.)

Green Chili and Cheese Cornbread Muffins

TEXTURE: REGULAR

These muffins are perfect with soup or chili.

½ cup (55 g) all-purpose flour

½ cup (70 g) coarse yellow cornmeal

1 teaspoon baking powder

½ teaspoon baking soda

¼ teaspoon salt

1½ teaspoon onion powder

½ cup (120 ml) low-fat buttermilk

1 egg

2 tablespoons (12 g) diced mild green chilies, drained

½ cup (55 g) reduced-fat shredded Cheddar cheese

—

Yield: Makes 8 (2-ounce) muffins

Preheat the oven to 400°F (200°C, or gas mark 6). Spray a muffin tin with cooking spray.

In a large mixing bowl, combine the flour, cornmeal, baking powder, baking soda, salt, and onion powder. Stir to combine.

In a medium mixing bowl, whisk together the buttermilk, egg, chiles, and cheese, just enough to combine. (The batter should be slightly lumpy.)

Fill 8 of the muffin cups two-thirds full with batter. Bake for 20 to 25 minutes, until a toothpick inserted into the middle of a muffin comes out clean. Let the muffins cool for 15 minutes before turning the tin over to release the muffins. (If the muffins stick to the pan, a slight tap on the back should help to release them.)

NUTRITIONAL ANALYSIS

EACH WITH: Calories: 93.10, Protein: 4.35 g, Carbs: 13.36 g, Total Fat: 2.43 g, Sat Fat: 1.17 g, Cholesterol: 34.36 mg, Sodium: 254.99 mg, Sugars: 1.09 g, Fiber: 0.92 g

Bacon-Cheddar Muffins

TEXTURE: REGULAR

You can't go wrong with the flavors of bacon and cheese. To save time, prepare the bacon strips per the package instructions, then chop or break them into crumbles.

½ cup (55 g) all-purpose flour

½ cup (70 g) coarse yellow cornmeal

1 teaspoon baking powder

½ teaspoon baking soda

⅛ teaspoon salt

½ cup (120 ml) low-fat buttermilk

1 egg

2 tablespoons (15 g) chopped green onion

½ cup (55 g) reduced-fat shredded Cheddar cheese

¼ cup (20 g) turkey bacon crumbles, prepared as per package instructions (about 4 strips)

—
Yield: Makes 8 (2-ounce) muffins

Preheat the oven to 375°F (190°C, or gas mark 5). Spray a muffin tin with cooking spray.

In a large mixing bowl, combine the flour, cornmeal, baking powder, baking soda, and salt. Stir to combine.

In a medium mixing bowl, whisk together the buttermilk, egg, green onion, cheese, and bacon, just enough to combine. (The batter should be slightly lumpy.)

Fill 8 of the muffin cups two-thirds full with batter. Bake for 20 to 25 minutes, until a toothpick inserted into the middle of a muffin comes out clean. Let the muffins cool for 15 minutes before turning the tin over to release the muffins. (If the muffins stick to the pan, a slight tap on the back should help to release them.)

NUTRITIONAL ANALYSIS

EACH WITH: Calories: 101.19, Protein: 5.47 g, Carbs: 12.34 g, Total Fat: 3.65 g, Sat Fat: 1.38 g, Cholesterol: 39.36 mg, Sodium: 380.42 mg, Sugars: 0.91 g, Fiber: 1.01 g

Curried Carrot Soup

TEXTURE: PUREED. MAY BE CONSIDERED FULL LIQUID BY SOME MEAL PROGRAMS

"The carrot soup was absolutely delicious!"

—Mary Kate, *a gastric bypass patient in the Boston area*

3 pounds (1.5 kg) carrots, peeled and cut into 2-inch (5-cm) pieces

1 large russet potato, diced into ½-inch (1.25-cm) pieces

4 quarts (4 L) water

1 large yellow onion, diced into ¼-inch (6-mm) pieces

4 quarts (4 L) low-sodium vegetable broth

3 tablespoons (20 g) curry powder

2 teaspoon cayenne pepper (optional)

1 teaspoon cinnamon

1 teaspoon ground coriander seed

¼ cup (60 ml) lemon juice

Paprika

—
Yield: Makes 5 (1-cup) servings

In a 6-quart (6-L) soup pot, place the carrots, potato, and water. Bring to a boil, and then add the onion. Continue cooking for 12 to 15 minutes, until the carrots and potatoes are soft throughout. Drain in a colander, reserving half the liquid in a separate container, and set aside. Place the carrot mixture in a food processor fitted with a metal S blade and puree. (You may need to do this in batches.)

Return the pureed mixture to the soup pot. Add the broth, curry powder, cayenne pepper (if using), cinnamon, coriander, and lemon juice. Stir the mixture until an even consistency is reached. Cover and simmer over low heat for about 30 minutes. If a thinner consistency is desired, slowly add the reserved liquid from the carrots and potatoes until the desired consistency is reached. (The more liquid you add, the weaker the flavor becomes.) Serve in warmed bowls with a pinch of paprika sprinkled over the top for garnish.

NUTRITIONAL ANALYSIS

EACH WITH: Calories: 233.64, Protein: 8.18 g, Carbs: 49.37 g, Total Fat: 1.45 g, Sat Fat: 0.23 g, Cholesterol: 0.00 mg, Sodium: 387.76 mg, Sugars: 14.63 g, Fiber: 11.51 g

Green Tomato Soup with Fresh Tarragon

TEXTURE: PUREED. MAY BE CONSIDERED FULL LIQUID BY SOME MEAL PROGRAMS

Here's a great way to use the green tomatoes left on the summer gardener's vines.

1 tablespoon (14 ml) extra-virgin olive oil

Olive-oil-flavored cooking spray

3 cups (480 g) diced yellow onion

8 medium green tomatoes, cored and chopped into 1-inch (2.5-cm) pieces

2 teaspoons coriander seed

2½ teaspoons fresh tarragon leaves

2 cups (475 ml) natural low-sodium chicken broth

Salt (optional)

½ teaspoon fresh cracked black pepper

¼ cup (50 g) nonfat sour cream or nonfat plain yogurt (optional)

4 sprigs fresh tarragon

In a 6-quart (6-L) stockpot or Dutch oven, heat the oil and cooking spray over medium-high heat. Add the onion, tomatoes, coriander, tarragon leaves, salt (if using), and pepper. Sauté the mixture, stirring just enough to expose all ingredients to the heat surface. Continue to sauté until soft, but do not brown. Remove the pot from the heat and let the mixture cool for 10 minutes.

Place the mixture into a food processor fitted with metal S blade or blender and pulse until almost pureed consistency. Return the mixture to the pot and add the broth. Bring to a simmer, cover, and continue simmering for 20 minutes. Check the seasoning and adjust with salt if necessary. Serve in warmed soup bowls with a dollop of sour cream or yogurt (if using) and the tarragon sprigs.

—
Yield: Makes 5 (1-cup) servings

NUTRITIONAL ANALYSIS

EACH WITH: Calories: 123.29, Protein: 4.64 g, Carbs: 20.81 g, Total Fat: 3.42 g, Sat Fat: 0.49 g, Cholesterol: 0.00 mg, Sodium: 220.90 mg, Sugars: 11.98 g, Fiber: 3.87 g,

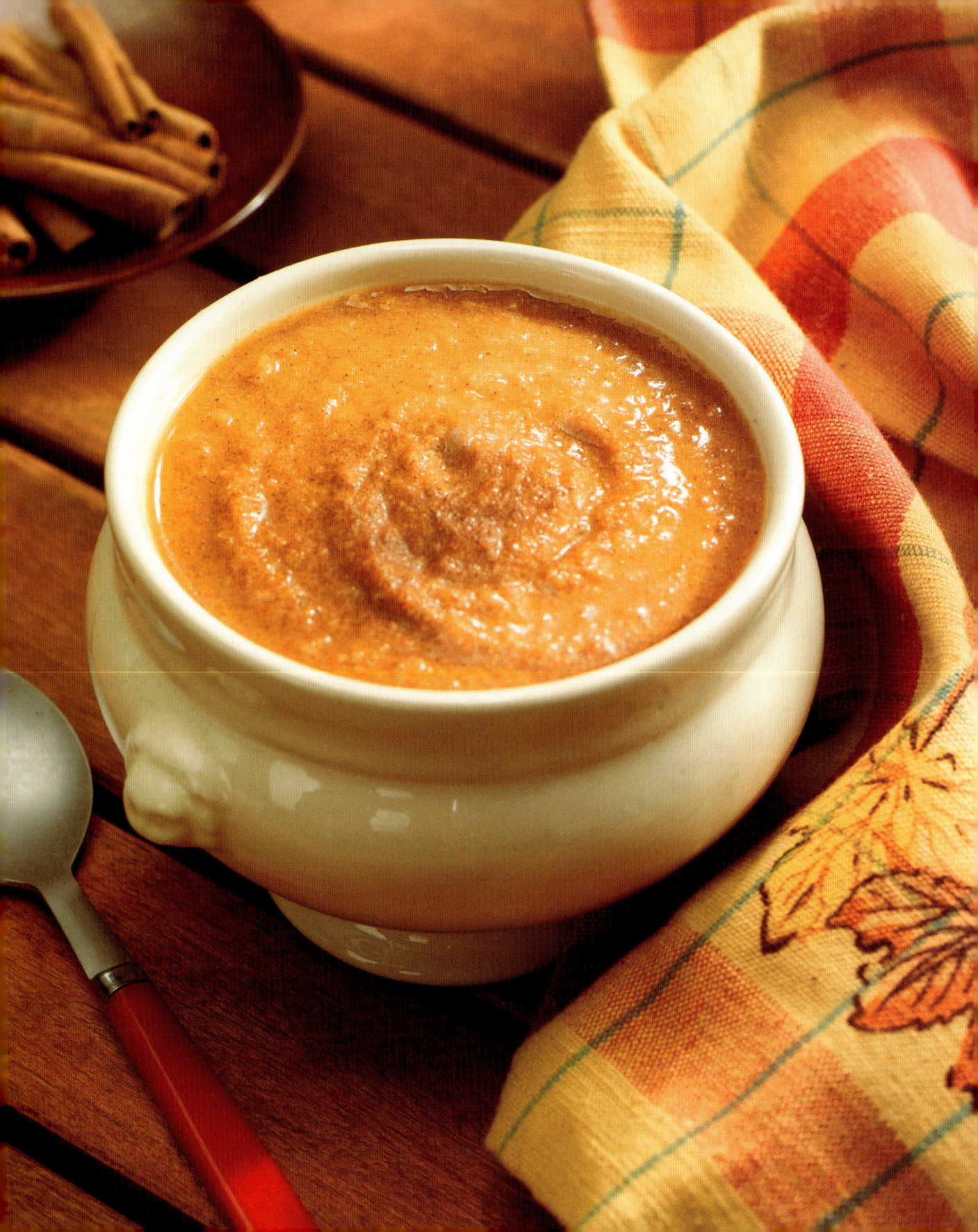

Fall Harvest Pumpkin Soup

TEXTURE: PUREED

This soup is delicious, fun, and a great source of vitamin A. Include the curry powder and cayenne pepper if you like a lot of heat.

3 cups (735 g) pureed canned pumpkin (no salt) or 1 (5-pound, or 2.5 kg) sugar pumpkin

1 large yellow onion, diced

2 large celery ribs cut into ½-inch (1.25-cm) pieces

1 quart (1 L) low-sodium chicken stock

½ cup (120 ml) white wine, cooking sherry, chicken broth, or vegetable broth

2 teaspoons cinnamon, plus more for garnish (optional)

2 teaspoons allspice

2 teaspoons curry powder (optional)

2 teaspoons paprika

½ teaspoon cumin

1 teaspoon cayenne pepper (optional)

½ teaspoon ground white pepper

¾ cup (175 ml) nonfat half-and-half (see note)

—
Yield: Makes 6 (1-cup) servings

MARGARET'S NOTE

If you use light half-and-half instead of nonfat, the sugar content will increase to 9 grams per serving, which is still within the 14 grams or less per serving as my general recommendation for weight-loss surgery patients. However, if you use low-sugar, the sugar content will decrease to 3 grams per serving. The taste difference may or may not be noticeable, depending on your individual preferences. Either one is nutritionally acceptable.

If using fresh pumpkin, preheat the oven to 375°F (190°C, or gas mark 5).

Cut the pumpkin in half and scrape out the seed and strings. Cut the halves into quarters. Place the pumpkin, skin-side down, in a 9½- x 13½-inch (22.5- x 32.5-cm) or 3-quart (3-L) baking dish, with about ½ inch (1.25 cm) of water in it. Bake the pumpkin for about 60 minutes, until the flesh is tender throughout. Let it cool and scrape out the flesh.

Puree the pumpkin using a hand mixer, blender, or food processor. (You'll have about 3 cups puree.)

In a 4-quart (4-L) soup pot, place the chicken stock, onion, and celery. Cover and bring it to a simmer. Continue cooking for about 15 minutes, until the vegetables are soft and translucent. With a slotted spoon or small mesh strainer, remove the vegetables and puree, using the same method as the pumpkin. Return the vegetables to the chicken stock and add the pumpkin puree. Add the wine (or sherry or broth), cinnamon, allspice, curry powder (if using), paprika, cumin, cayenne pepper (if using), and white pepper. Slowly stir in the half-and-half. Bring it back to a simmer and continue cooking for about 20 minutes, stirring occasionally. Serve in warmed soup bowls, and garnish with a light sprinkle of cinnamon (if using).

NUTRITIONAL ANALYSIS

EACH WITH: Calories: 151.17, Protein: 5.82 g, Carbs: 21.99 g, Total Fat: 3.58 g, Sat Fat: 0.72 g, Cholesterol: 4.54 mg, Sodium: 252.18 mg, Sugars: 7.44 g, Fiber: 5.13 g,

Lentil Soup

TEXTURE: SOFT

Rich in fiber, protein, and iron, this soup is tasty, too.

1 tablespoon (14 ml) extra-virgin olive oil

1 cup (130 g) diced carrot (about 1 large)

¾ cup (120 g) diced yellow onion
(about 1 medium)

1 cup (100 g) diced celery (about 1 large rib)

2 cloves fresh garlic, chopped

2 bay leaves

1 tablespoon (14 ml) low-sodium tamari soy sauce

½ teaspoon black pepper

1 teaspoon dried oregano

1 teaspoon dried thyme

1 can (14.5 ounces, or 415 g) plum tomatoes,
drained

2 cups (385 g) green lentils, s
oaked for 30 minutes (see note)

4½ cups (1 L) water

Water or low-sodium vegetable broth (optional)

6 sprigs fresh thyme

—

Yield: Makes about 6 (1-cup) servings

In a 3-quart (3-L) stockpot or soup pot over medium-high heat, heat the oil. Add the carrot, onion, celery, garlic, bay leaves, tamari soy sauce, pepper, oregano, and dried thyme, and cook until the carrots begin to soften. Break apart the tomatoes by crushing them with your hands, then add them to the pot. Drain the lentils and then add them to the pot. Add the water and bring to a boil. Reduce the heat to a soft boil, cover partially, and cook for 20 minutes, until the lentils become soft throughout. If a thinner consistency is desired, add additional water or low-sodium vegetable broth in small amounts at a time. (Adding too much water to the soup will decrease the strength in flavor.) Remove the bay leaves prior to serving. Garnish with the thyme sprigs and serve in warmed soup bowls.

NUTRITIONAL ANALYSIS

EACH WITH: Calories: 312.58, Protein: 20.20 g, Carbs: 48.78 g, Total Fat: 4.91 g, Sat Fat: 1.04 g, Cholesterol: 0.00 mg, Sodium: 393.70 mg, Sugars: 10.79 g, Fiber: 23.14 g

MARGARET'S NOTE

Although lentils are high in protein, they need to be soaked for at least 30 minutes to help remove the phytates (natural mineral binders) that might impede the absorption of iron.

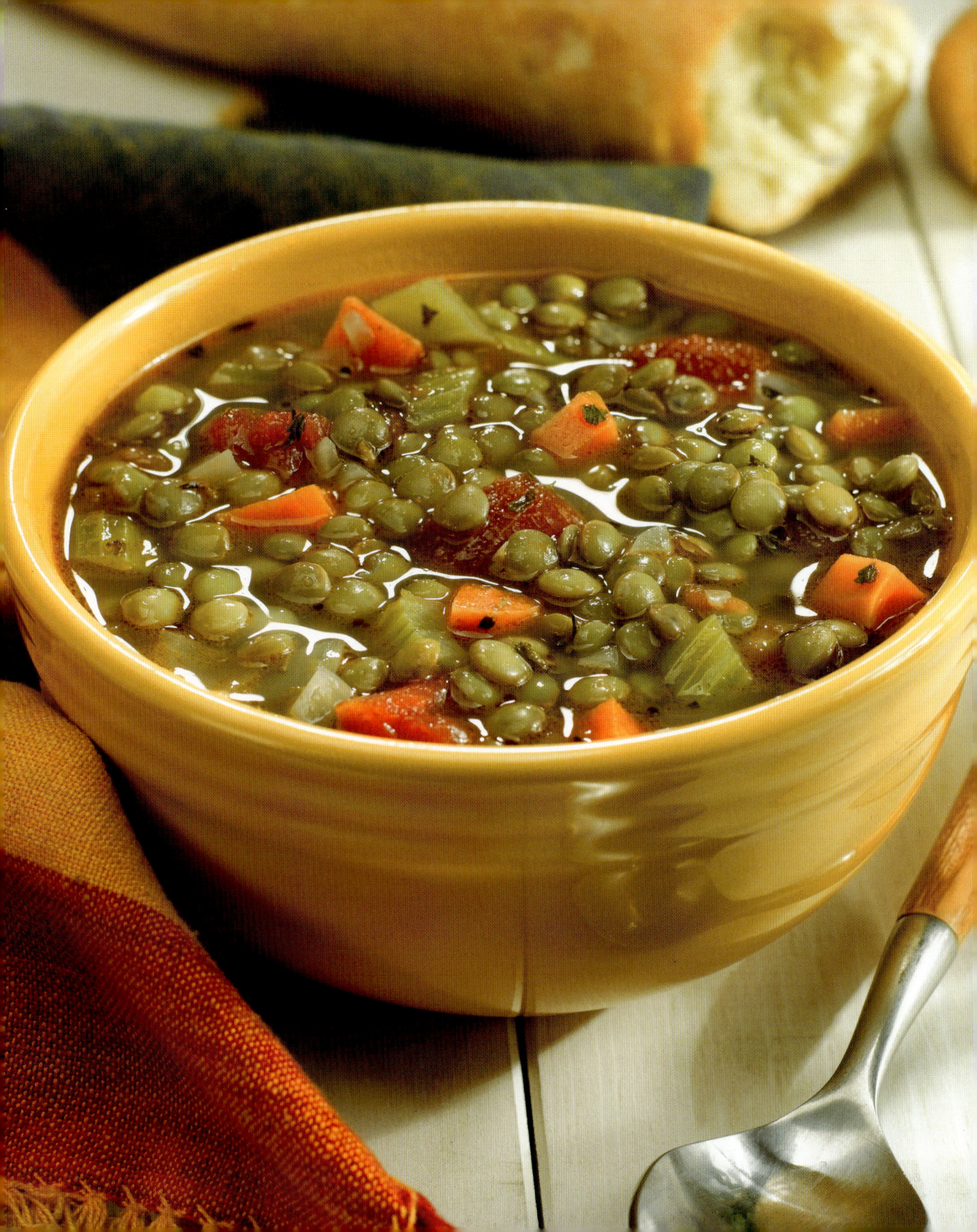

Creamy Tomato Parmesan Soup

TEXTURE: PUREED

1 cup (150 g) peeled and diced Yukon Gold potatoes (about 1 large potato)

½ cup (80 g) diced yellow onion (about ½ large onion)

2 cloves garlic, chopped

½ teaspoon basil

½ teaspoon oregano

¼ teaspoon black pepper

¼ teaspoon salt

2 cans (14.5 ounces, or 415 g each) diced tomatoes in juice (no salt added)

½ cups (120 ml) 2% milk

¼ cup (60 ml) plain low-fat yogurt

2 tablespoons (10 g) grated Parmesan cheese

1 tablespoon (4 g) chopped fresh parsley

—

Yield: Makes 4 (1- cup) servings

In a 2-quart (2-L) saucepan, place the potatoes, onion, garlic, basil, oregano, pepper, and salt with enough water to cover 1 inch (2.5 cm) above the level of the vegetables. Bring to a boil, then reduce the heat and simmer uncovered for about 15 minutes, until the potatoes are tender throughout.

Drain the tomatoes, reserving the juice. Place the tomatoes in a food processor or blender and puree. Add the tomatoes and juice to the saucepan.

In a separate 4-cup (1-L) mixing bowl, mix the milk, yogurt, and cheese, stirring until a smooth consistency is reached.

Bring the soup to a simmer and slowly add the yogurt-milk mixture, stirring vigorously with a wire whip until all ingredients are evenly incorporated. Serve in warmed soup bowls and garnish with the parsley.

NUTRITIONAL ANALYSIS

EACH WITH: Calories: 92.39, Protein: 6.82 g, Carbs: 15.21 g, Total Fat: 1.36 g, Sat Fat: 0.80 g, Cholesterol: 4.75 mg, Sodium: 363.65 mg, Sugars: 8.24 g, Fiber: 2.63 g

Black Bean Soup

High in fiber, this is super tasty, too!

½ cup (90 g) long-grain brown rice, raw, rinsed, and drained

1 cup (235 ml) water

2 cans (16 ounces, or 455 g each) black beans, drained

1 tablespoon (14 ml) olive oil

1 medium onion, diced

1 tablespoon (6 g) finely chopped jalapeño pepper

2 cloves garlic, minced

1½ teaspoons ground cumin

½ teaspoon cayenne pepper (optional)

1 teaspoon oregano

1 teaspoon paprika

1 teaspoon chili powder

1 can (11 ounces, or 310 g) diced tomatoes, drained

1½ quarts (1.5 L) low-sodium chicken broth

Juice of ½ fresh lime

2 tablespoons (2 g) chopped fresh cilantro

1 cup (115 g) reduced-fat shredded Cheddar cheese

—

Yield: Makes 8 (about 1-cup) servings

In a 1-quart (1-L) saucepan, place the rice and water and bring to a boil.

Immediately reduce the heat to a simmer, then loosely cover and simmer for about 15 minutes, until all the liquid is absorbed. Remove from the heat.

In a food processor, puree the beans and set aside.

In a 3-quart (3-L) saucepan, heat the oil over medium-high heat. Add the onion, jalapeno, garlic, cumin, cayenne pepper (if using), oregano, paprika, and chili powder and sauté until the onion begins to soften. Add the tomatoes and stir. Add the pureed beans, rice, broth, and lime juice and stir with a wire whip. Bring to a soft simmer and continue cooking for 20 minutes, stirring once every 5 minutes. Serve in warmed soup bowls and garnish with the cilantro and cheese.

NUTRITIONAL ANALYSIS

EACH WITH: Calories: 206.02, Protein: 11.28 g, Carbs: 29.66 g, Total Fat: 4.38 g, Sat Fat: 2.21 g, Cholesterol: 10.00 mg, Sodium: 535.08 mg, Sugars: 2.51 g, Fiber: 5.76 g

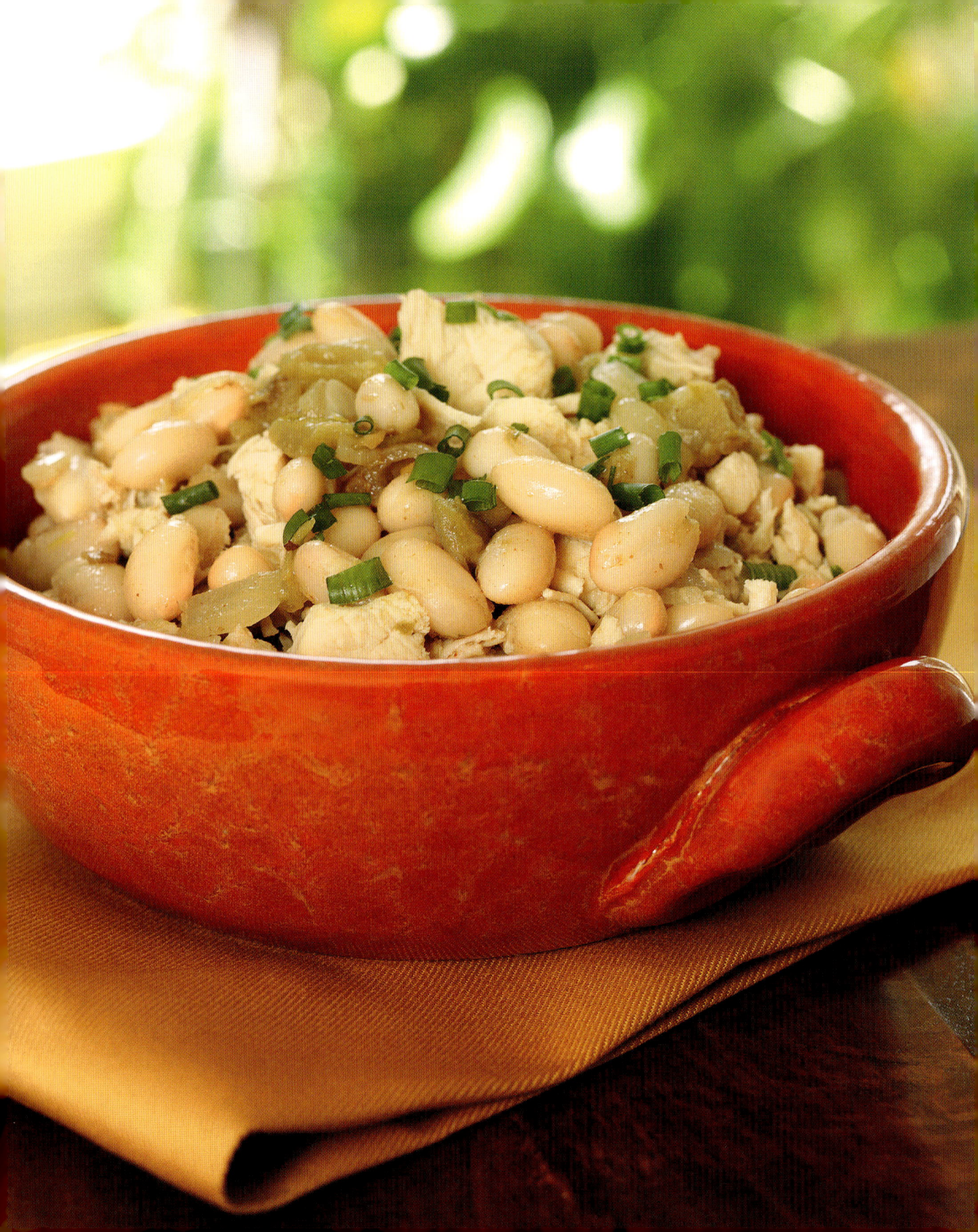

White Chicken Chili

This is a wonderful recipe contributed by a Baltimore woman named Teresa who is having an amazingly successful journey after gastric bypass surgery. This is so quick and easy, you won't believe it!

1 tablespoon (15 ml) canola oil

1½ cups (240 g) chopped white onion

2 cans (4 ounces, or 113 g each) chopped green chile peppers

1 teaspoon dried oregano

1 teaspoon ground cumin

1 teaspoon ground cumin

¼ teaspoon cayenne pepper

2 cans (15 ounces, or 425 g each) great northern beans, rinsed and drained

4 cups (946 ml) reduced-sodium chicken broth

4 cups (560 g) diced cooked chicken breast

2 tablespoons (30 ml) apple cider vinegar

—

Yield: Makes 14 (1-cup) servings

Heat the canola oil in a large pot or Dutch oven over medium-high heat. Add the onion and cook, stirring occasionally, until softened, about 5 minutes.

Stir in the chiles, oregano, cumin, and cayenne. Cook, stirring occasionally, for 5 minutes.

Stir in the beans and broth, and bring to a simmer. Cook, stirring occasionally, for 20 minutes.

Add the chicken and vinegar; cook for 5 minutes more.

NUTRITIONAL ANALYSIS

EACH WITH: Calories: 153.62, Protein: 23.36 g, Carbs: 11.72 g, Total Fat: 25.23 g, Sat Fat: 3.75 g, Cholesterol: 54.79 mg, Sodium: 783.72 mg, Sugars: 2.72 g, Fiber: 4.01 g

Potato Leek Soup with Fresh Tarragon

TEXTURE: PUREED

1½ to 2 cups (225 to 300 g) peeled and diced russet potatoes

1¾ pounds (795 g) leeks (2 large or 3 medium)

2 tablespoons (28 g) margarine or light butter (see note)

2 cloves garlic, minced

1 teaspoon black pepper

5 cups (40 ounces, or 1185 ml) low-sodium chicken broth

¼ cup (15 g) fresh, coarsely chopped tarragon leaves

4 to 6 whole tarragon sprigs (optional)

—
Yield: Makes 5 (about 1-cup) servings

LYNETTE'S NOTE

Try to find a light margarine or butter that has the same consistency and flavor as real butter. It may cost a bit more, but there are some good substitutes available.

In a 2-quart (2-L) saucepan, cover the potatoes with water and bring it to a boil. Continue cooking for about 12 minutes, until the potatoes are tender throughout. Remove from the heat and drain in a colander. Set aside.

Cut the green tops away from the leeks and discard them. Split the white portions of the leeks down the middle, leaving just the roots intact, and wash them clean of all sand and grit. Drain in a colander. Slice the leeks into thin half-coins. Discard the roots and set aside.

In a 4-quart (4-L) soup pot, melt the margarine over medium heat. Add the leeks, garlic, and pepper and cook until the leeks are tender, but not brown. Add the broth, potatoes, and tarragon leaves and bring to a simmer over low heat. Cook for about 15 minutes. Remove from the heat and let cool for about 15 minutes. With a slotted spoon, remove three-quarters of the solid ingredients and place in a blender or food processor. Blend until smooth. Return the mixture to the soup pot. Heat and stir to an even consistency. Serve in warmed soup bowls and garnish with the tarragon sprigs (if using).

NUTRITIONAL ANALYSIS

EACH WITH: Calories: 186.63, Protein: 5.24 g, Carbs: 36.71 g, Total Fat: 3.05 g, Sat Fat: 0.51 g, Cholesterol: 0.00 mg, Sodium: 96.93 mg, Sugars: 6.73 g, Fiber: 4.57 g

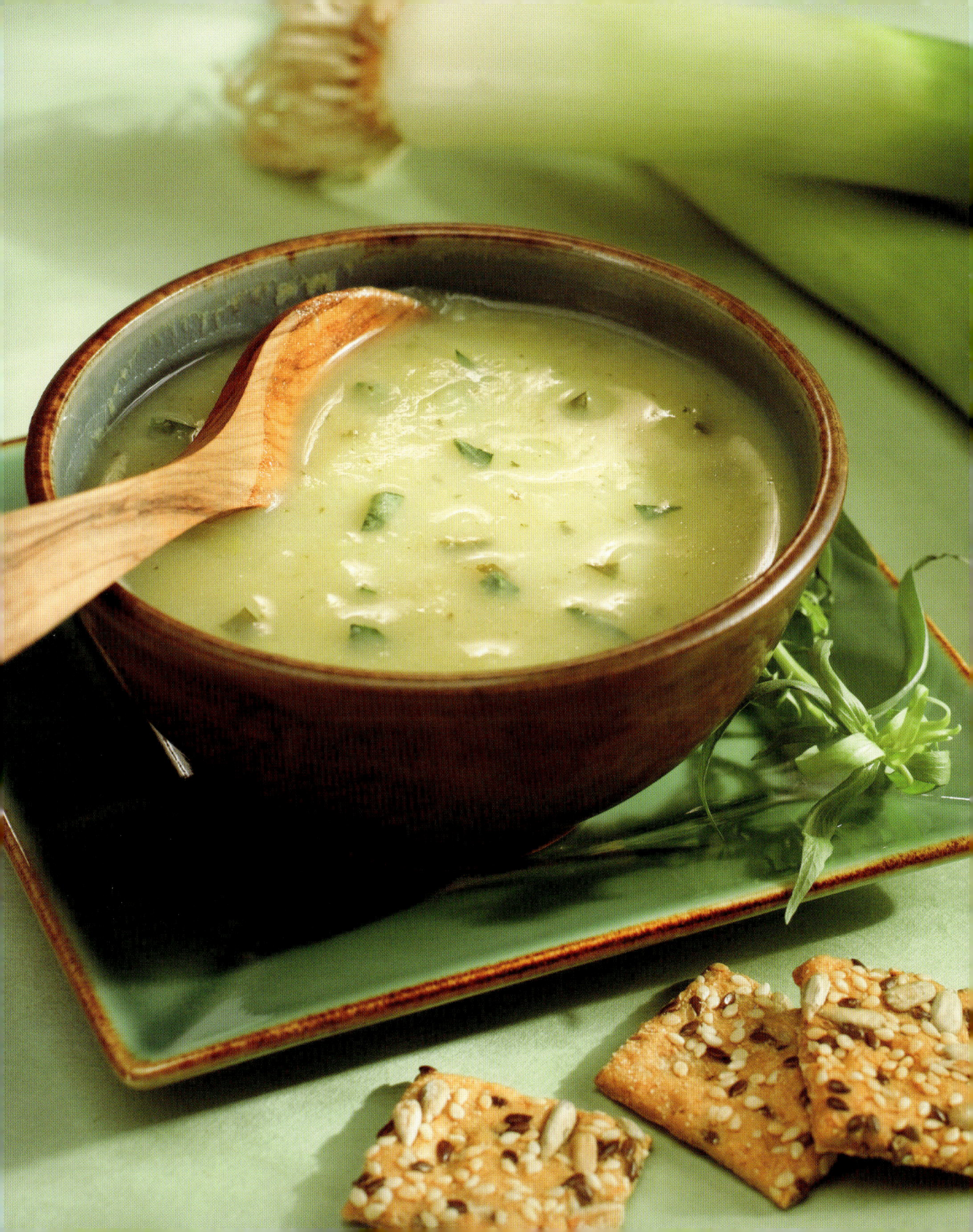

Chicken and Sausage Gumbo

TEXTURE: REGULAR

You're going to love this zesty gumbo! It's packed full of flavor and protein.

1 bag (3½ ounces, or 45 g) boil-in-bag brown rice

2 tablespoons (16 g) whole-wheat flour

1 tablespoon (15 ml) extra-virgin olive oil

1 medium onion, chopped

2 medium bell peppers, chopped

1 cup (227 g) frozen okra

1 cup (100 g) chopped celery

2 cloves garlic, chopped

½ teaspoon dried thyme

¼ teaspoon paprika

2 cups (280 g) chopped cooked chicken breast

4 ounces (55 g) turkey kielbasa, cut into ½-inch (1.25-cm) pieces

1 can (14½ ounces, or 411 g) low-sodium diced tomatoes with peppers and onions

1 can (14½ ounces, or 440 ml) fat-free, low-sodium chicken broth

—

Yield: Makes 6 (about 1-cup) servings

Prepare the rice according to the package instructions, minus the salt and fat.

While the rice is cooking, combine the flour and oil in a Dutch oven or large heavy-duty pot. Sauté over medium-high heat, stirring constantly, for 3 minutes. Add the onion, bell peppers, okra, celery, garlic, thyme, and paprika. Cook for about 3 minutes, or until the vegetables are tender.

Stir in the chicken, kielbasa, tomatoes, and broth. Cook for 6 more minutes, or until thoroughly heated. Serve over the brown rice.

NUTRITIONAL ANALYSIS

EACH WITH: Calories: 265.51, Protein: 22.52 g, Carbs: 24.68 g, Total Fat: 8.25 g, Sat Fat: 1.96 g, Cholesterol: 61.61 mg, Sodium: 613.06 mg, Sugars: 5.30 g, Fiber: 3.35 g

Julianna's Kale, Apple, and Lentil Soup

TEXTURE: MECHANICAL SOFT

This delicious recipe, from Julianna Pax, Ph.D., shows just how versatile lentils can be. Try this recipe, and the other Lentil Soup, found on page 50, to see which flavor suits your fancy.

1 pound (454 g) green lentils, picked over and rinsed

6 cups (1419 ml) low-sodium chicken broth

8 cups (1892 ml) water

2 cups (320 g) chopped white onion

2 cups (260 g) peeled and chopped carrots

1¼ cups (111 g) washed and sliced leeks

1 teaspoon dried thyme or poultry seasoning

4 cups (268 g) chopped kale, stems removed

2 tablespoons (30 ml) canola oil

3 cups (375 g) peeled and chopped apple

1 teaspoon salt

½ teaspoon ground black pepper

—

Yield: Makes 16 (about 1-cup) servings

In a 10-quart (10-L) soup pot, add the lentils, broth, and water. Bring to a boil, then simmer, covered, for 30 minutes. As soon as you have the onions and carrots chopped, add them to the simmering pot. Cover the pot and continue simmering for another 30 minutes.

Add the leeks, thyme or poultry seasoning, and kale to the pot and continue simmering, covered, for 10 to 15 more minutes.

In a separate pan, heat the canola oil over medium-high heat. Add the apples. Season with salt and pepper and sauté for 4 to 5 minutes, or until the apples are golden on all sides. Add the apples to the lentil mixture.

NUTRITIONAL ANALYSIS

EACH WITH: Calories: 138.22, Protein: 7.92 g, Carbs: 26.78 g, Total Fat: 0.89 g Sat Fat 0.04 g, Cholesterol: 0.00 mg, Sodium: 338.04 mg, Sugars: 4.96 g, Fiber: 6.36 g

Whole-Wheat Elbow Macaroni Salad

TEXTURE: REGULAR

Bring this pasta salad to a potluck or barbecue. Garnish it with fresh tomato wedges.

1 cup (105 g) dry whole-wheat macaroni

½ cup (115 g) nonfat mayonnaise

1 teaspoon Dijon mustard

1 tablespoon (14 ml) lemon juice

1 teaspoon celery salt

½ teaspoon black pepper

½ cup (80 g) finely chopped red onion

¾ cup (75 g) finely chopped celery

½ cup (70 g) finely chopped red bell pepper

1 tablespoon (9 g) sliced black olives

1 tablespoon (4 g) chopped fresh parsley

1½ teaspoons finely chopped green onion

—

Yield: Makes about 8 (½-cup) servings

Cook the macaroni according to package instructions, omitting the salt and oil. Drain the macaroni and cool completely in the refrigerator.

While the macaroni cools, place the mayonnaise, mustard, lemon juice, celery salt, and pepper in a small mixing bowl and stir to combine.

When the pasta is completely cooled, place it in a large mixing bowl along with the onion, celery, bell pepper, olives, parsley, and green onion and pour the dressing over the top. Using a large spoon or rubber spatula, gently stir the pasta until it is completely covered with dressing. Transfer to a serving bowl.

NUTRITIONAL ANALYSIS

EACH WITH: Calories: 69.92, Protein: 2.41 g, Carbs: 14.32 g, Total Fat: 0.51 g, Sat Fat: 0.05 g, Cholesterol: 0.01 mg, Sodium: 156.99 mg, Sugars: 3.14 g, Fiber: 1.96 g

Classic Spinach Salad with Apple Cider Vinaigrette

TEXTURE: REGULAR

This can be served as a side salad or an entrée. It's perfect for a light summer dinner. Make the dressing at least 20 minutes ahead of time. It's great topped with toasted slivered almonds.

2 tablespoons (28 ml) olive oil

1 tablespoon (14 ml) apple cider vinegar

1 tablespoon (14 ml) fresh lemon juice

1 medium clove fresh garlic, cut into thin slivers

½ teaspoon low-sodium soy sauce

¼ teaspoon black pepper

8⅛-inch- (3-mm-) thick red onion rings

8 cups (240 g) fresh baby spinach, washed and thoroughly drained and dried

4 strips turkey bacon, cooked crisp and crumbled

1 small cucumber, peeled and thinly sliced

4 Italian plum tomatoes, cored and cut into 4 wedges each

2 hard-boiled eggs, cooled, peeled, and cut into 4 wedges each

—
Yield: Makes 8 (½-cup) servings or 4 (1 cup) servings

In a glass jar with a tightly fitting lid, place the oil, vinegar, lemon juice, garlic, soy sauce, and pepper. Shake vigorously. Set aside.

About 20 minutes before serving, place the onion in the jar of salad dressing to marinate.

In a large mixing bowl, place the spinach, bacon, and cucumber.

Remove the onion from the dressing and set aside. Pour the dressing evenly over the salad and gently toss, just enough to ensure complete coverage. Distribute the dressed salad evenly in the center of 4 entrée plates or 8 side salad plates. Place the tomato wedges leaning against the outer edges of each salad. Place the egg wedges next to the tomato wedges. Top the salads with 1 or 2 onion rings. Serve immediately.

NUTRITIONAL ANALYSIS

EACH WITH: Calories: 90.46, Protein: 3.86 g, Carbs: 5.79 g, Total Fat: 6.10 g, Sat Fat: 1.14 g, Cholesterol: 65.00 mg, Sodium: 163.85 mg, Sugars: 2.11 g, Fiber: 1.80 g

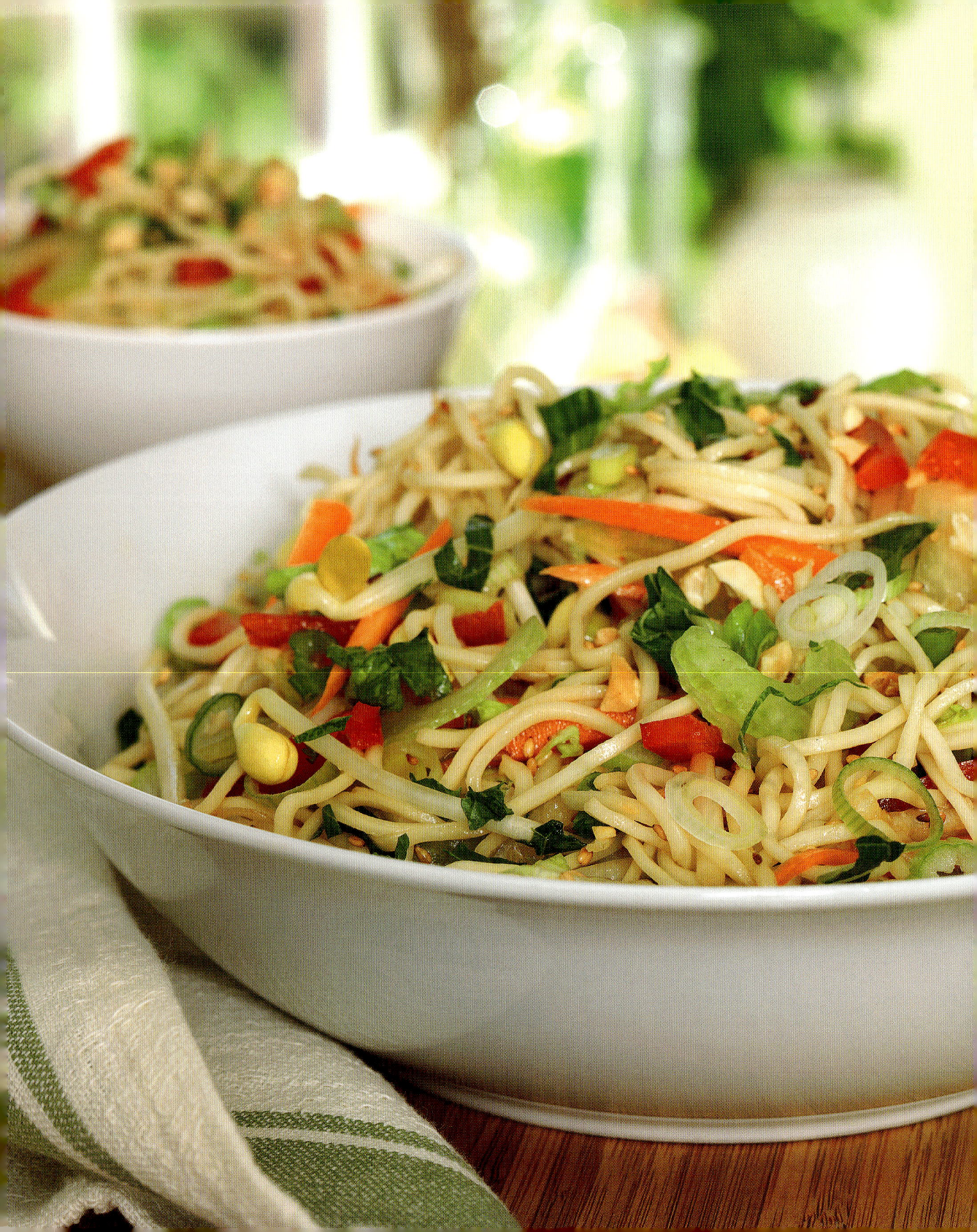

Asian Noodle Salad

TEXTURE: REGULAR

This yummy recipe comes from Teresa, a gastric bypass surgery patient in Baltimore.

1 package (12 ounces, or 210 g) soba noodles or whole-wheat noodles

1 teaspoon sesame oil

2 tablespoons (30 ml) rice wine vinegar

3 tablespoons (45 ml) low-sodium soy sauce

1 teaspoon hot chili oil

1 tablespoon (16 ml) hoisin sauce

3 tablespoons (45 ml) extra-virgin olive oil

1 carrot, thinly sliced or julienned

2 celery stalks, thinly sliced or julienned

5 scallions, white and light green parts, thinly sliced

½ cup (45 g) thinly sliced napa cabbage

½ red bell pepper, thinly sliced or julienned

½ cup (45 g) julienned bok choy

1 cup (50 g) bean sprouts, optional

3 tablespoons (3 g) fresh cilantro, minced

3 tablespoons (24 g) sesame seeds, toasted

2 tablespoons (18 g) unsalted peanuts, roughly chopped

—
Yield: Makes 8 (about ½-cup) servings

In a medium stock pot, cook the noodles according to the package directions. When finished, place the noodles in an ice-water bath to cool. Drain and set aside.

In a medium bowl combine the sesame oil, vinegar, soy sauce, hot chili oil, hoisin sauce, and olive oil. Add the carrot, celery, scallions, cabbage, bell pepper, bok choy, bean sprouts (if using), cilantro, and cooled noodles. Mix to combine. Garnish with sesame seeds and peanuts.

NUTRITIONAL ANALYSIS

EACH WITH: Calories: 280.73, Protein: 9.62 g, Carbs: 37.95 g, Total Fat: 10.41 g, Sat Fat: 1.11 g, Cholesterol: 0.00 mg, Sodium: 355.33 mg, Sugars: 5.87 g, Fiber: 3.50 g

Mandarin Pea Pod Salad

This salad is colorful, nutritious, and wonderful for home entertaining.

"This salad went over very well with us and our friends. The flavors were a great and refreshing combination."

—Jill and Dan, *gastric banding surgery patients in the Washington, D.C., area*

2 packages (10 ounces, 280 g each) prewashed fresh spinach

2 cups (475 ml) water

2 cups (about ¾ pound, 340 g) fresh snow peas

2 cups (500 g) canned mandarin oranges, drained

2 tablespoons (15 g) toasted sesame seeds (optional)

2 tablespoons (20 g) thinly sliced shallots

1 tablespoon (14 ml) extra-virgin olive oil

¼ cup (60 ml) apple cider vinegar

¼ teaspoon salt

¼ teaspoon black pepper

2 tablespoons (28 ml) fresh lime juice (from about ½ lime)

1 teaspoon lime zest (grated peel of about ½ lime)

—

Yield: Makes 8 (about ¾-cup) servings

Cut the stems off of the spinach and shred (with your hands) into about 1-inch (2.5-cm) pieces, arranging evenly on a serving platter.

In a 1½ -quart (1.5-L) saucepan, bring the water to a boil. Remove the stems and strings from the peas.

Prepare an ice bath by filling a medium mixing bowl with ice and just enough cold water to cover. Drop the peas into the boiling water and blanch them for about 45 seconds. With a strainer, remove the peas and immediately place them into the ice bath. (This stops the cooking process and helps to maintain beautiful, bright green color.) After 60 seconds in the ice bath, remove the peas, drain, pat dry with paper towels, and place evenly atop the spinach. Arrange the mandarin oranges evenly over the peas.

In a small plastic container with a lid, combine the sesame seeds (if using), shallots, oil, vinegar, salt, pepper, lime juice, and lime zest. Shake vigorously and/or whisk until the dressing is emulsified. Just prior to serving, pour the salad dressing evenly over the top.

NUTRITIONAL ANALYSIS

EACH WITH: Calories: 102.22, Protein: 3.49 g, Carbs: 17.09 g, Total Fat: 2.44 g, Sat Fat: 0.32 g, Cholesterol: 0.00 mg, Sodium: 99.57 mg, Sugars: 11.76 g, Fiber: 3.72 g

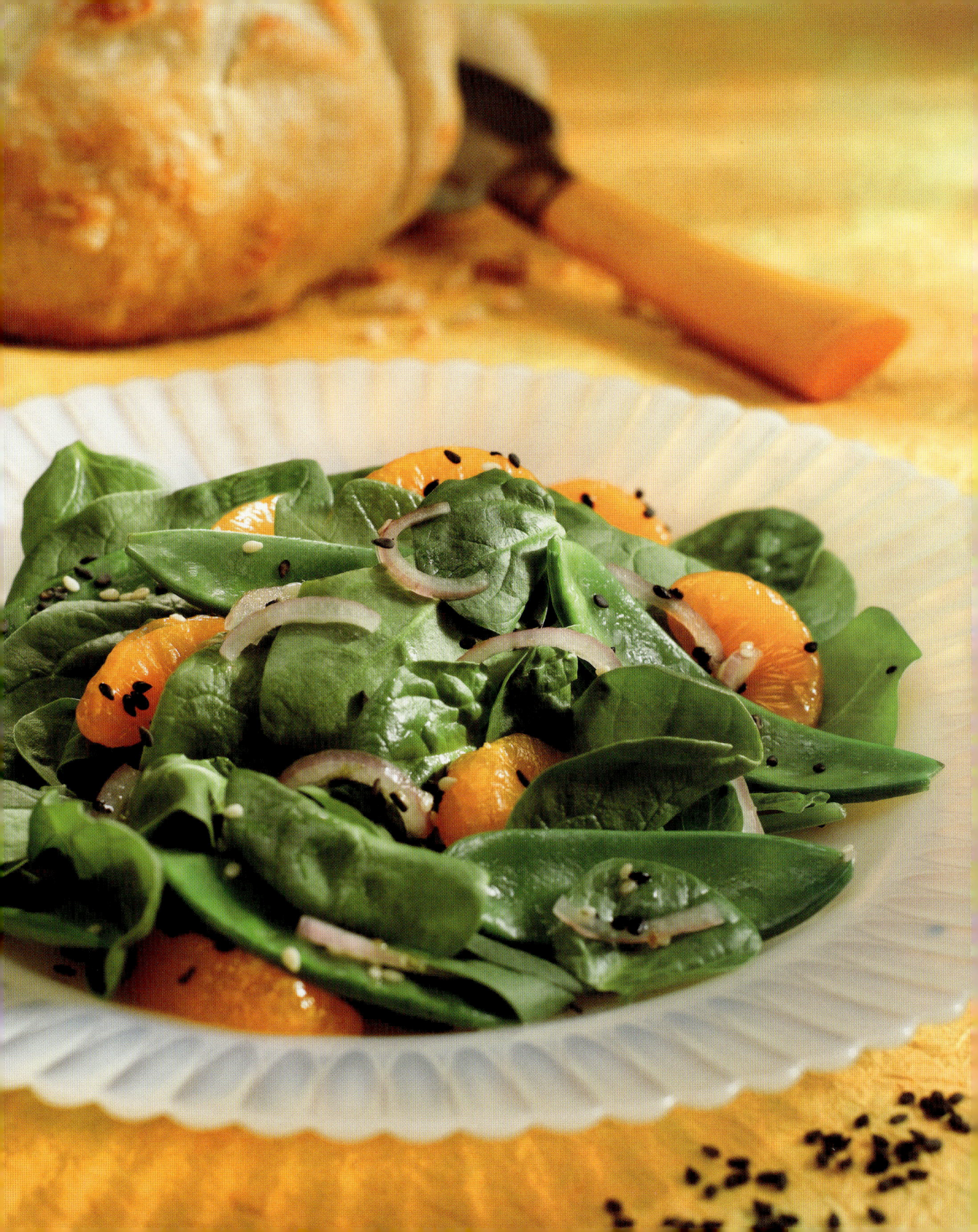

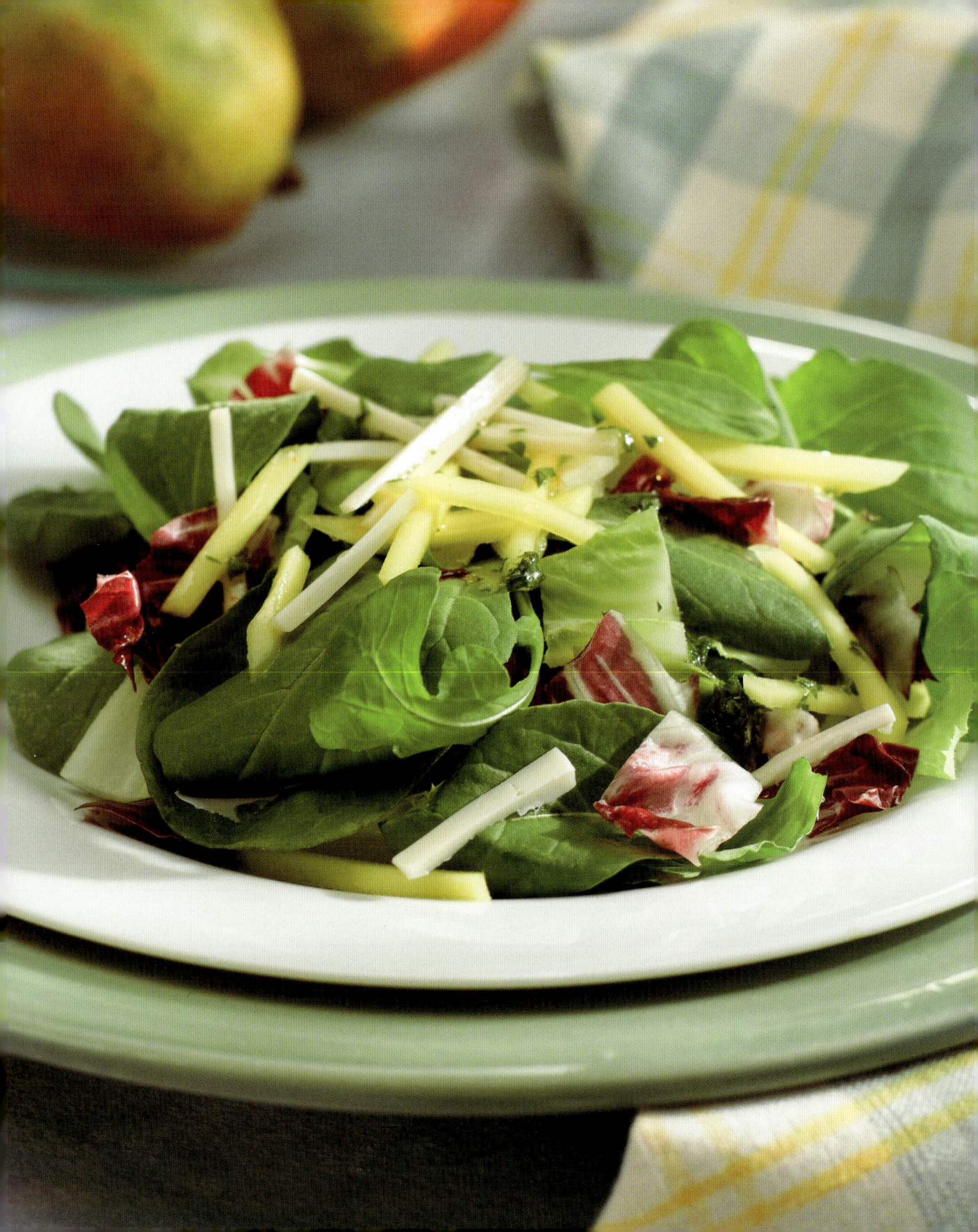

Hearts of Palm Salad with Arugula and Endive

TEXTURE: REGULAR

Try topping this salad with grilled chicken, shrimp, or pork tenderloin cut into thin strips.

Zest and juice of ½ lime

1 tablespoon (14 ml) apple cider vinegar

1 tablespoon (14 ml) fresh orange juice

⅛ teaspoon fresh minced garlic

Pinch cayenne pepper (optional)

2 tablespoons (28 ml) olive oil

3 teaspoons chopped fresh cilantro

3 cups (60 g) arugula, washed and dried

1 medium Belgium endive, cut into bite-size pieces

1 small radicchio, cut into bite-size pieces

4 stalks canned hearts of palm, cut into 1-inch (2.5-cm) match sticks

½ fresh mango, cut into about 1-inch (2.5-cm) strips

—

Yield: Makes 6 (about ¾-cup) servings

In a small mixing bowl, place the lime zest and lime juice. Add the vinegar, orange juice, garlic, and cayenne pepper (if using). Whisk with a wire whip to combine. Continue whisking while slowly adding the oil until the dressing is emulsified. Add the cilantro and stir. Set aside for the flavors to marry while preparing the salad.

In a salad bowl, place the arugula. Add the endive and radicchio. Top with the hearts of palm and mango. Toss with the dressing just before serving.

NUTRITIONAL ANALYSIS

EACH WITH: Calories: 87.56, Protein: 2.43 g, Carbs: 9.42 g, Total Fat: 5.16 g, Sat Fat: 0.78 g, Cholesterol: 0.00 mg, Sodium: 122.06 mg, Sugars: 3.67 g, Fiber: 3.93 g

Mexican Shrimp Salad with Jicama

TEXTURE: REGULAR

This south-of the-border salad combines shrimp with jicama, a refreshing flavor with a unique and crunchy texture.

⅓ cup (35 g) thinly sliced green onions

⅓ cup (75 g) nonfat mayonnaise

⅓ cup (80 g) nonfat plain yogurt

2 teaspoon red pepper sauce

1 tablespoon chopped fresh cilantro

2 teaspoons prepared horseradish

1 teaspoon chili powder

1 teaspoon ground cumin

2 teaspoons lime juice

1½ pounds (680 g) precooked medium-size shrimp

½ medium jicama, skinned and cut into about ½-inch (2.5-cm) pieces (about ¾ cup, or 90 g)

4 cups (80 g) hearty salad greens, ready to serve

2 tablespoons (28 ml) low-calorie Thousand Island dressing (prepared or on the next page)

—
Yield: Makes about 6 (1-cup) servings

In a medium mixing bowl, place the green onions, mayonnaise, yogurt, pepper sauce, cilantro, horseradish, chili powder, cumin, and lime juice and stir to combine. Add the shrimp and toss to cover with the dressing. Cover the bowl and refrigerate to marinate for 30 to 60 minutes. Add the jicama and stir to coat. Discard excess marinade.

In another medium mixing bowl, toss the salad greens with the Thousand Island dressing and shrimp. Serve on chilled salad plates.

NUTRITIONAL ANALYSIS

EACH WITH: Calories: 155.42, Protein: 24.34 g, Carbs: 8.22 g, Total Fat: 2.12 g, Sat Fat: 0.38 g, Cholesterol: 172.65 mg, Sodium: 365.22 mg, Sugars: 3.48 g, Fiber: 2.18 g

Thousand Island Dressing

TEXTURE: PUREED

1 cup (225 g) nonfat cottage cheese

⅓ cup (75 ml) low-fat buttermilk

1 teaspoon fresh lemon juice

2 tablespoons (30 g) sweet pickle relish

1 teaspoon red pepper sauce

1 tablespoon (15 g) low-carb ketchup

—

Yield: Makes 10 (about 2-tablespoon) servings

Place all of the ingredients in a blender or food processor and blend until smooth.

NUTRITIONAL ANALYSIS

EACH WITH: Calories: 24.20, Protein: 2.89 g, Carbs: 2.81 g, Total Fat: 0.09 g, Sat Fat: 0.05 g, Cholesterol: 1.33 mg, Sodium: 131.54 mg, Sugars: 1.62 g, Fiber: 0.04 g

Chickpea and Tomato Salad

TEXTURE: REGULAR

2 cans (15 ounces, or 425 g each) chickpeas, rinsed and dried

4 tomatoes, seeded and chopped

2 large hard-boiled eggs, peeled and chopped

2 cups (320 g) chopped Vidalia onion

3 tablespoons (45 ml) extra-virgin olive oil

⅓ cup (80 ml) white wine vinegar

1 teaspoon kosher salt

½ teaspoon black pepper

2 tablespoons (9 g) fresh parsley, chopped

—

Yield: Makes 8 (about 1-cup) servings

Combine the chickpeas, tomatoes, eggs, and onion in a large bowl.

In a smaller bowl, mix the olive oil, vinegar, salt, and pepper. Pour over the salad ingredients. Sprinkle with chopped parsley.

NUTRITIONAL ANALYSIS

EACH WITH: Calories: 188.98, Protein: 7.39 g, Carbs: 22.35 g, Total Fat: 8.31 g, Sat Fat: 1.13 g, Cholesterol: 53.75 mg, Sodium: 375.38 mg, Sugars: 6.16 g, Fiber: 5.33 g

Marinated Mushroom and Tomato Salad with Dijon Vinaigrette

TEXTURE: REGULAR

This salad is a great side dish for beef entrees.

1 pound (455 g) 1-inch (2.5-cm) button or crimini mushrooms

8 large ripe Roma tomatoes

¼ cup (40 g) thinly sliced red onion

¼ cup (60 ml) olive oil

1 tablespoon (14 ml) balsamic vinegar

1 teaspoon sugar

1 tablespoon (15 g) Dijon mustard

2 tablespoons (6 g) finely chopped fresh chives

½ teaspoon sea salt or kosher salt

¼ teaspoon fresh cracked black pepper

2 whole chive stems

—

Yield: Makes 12 (about ½-cup) servings

Clean the mushrooms with a mushroom brush or paper towels. Cut the end of the stems away and discard. Cut the mushrooms into halves.

Core the tomatoes and cut them in half lengthwise, then slice into ¼-inch (6 mm) half-circles.

In a medium mixing bowl, place the mushrooms, tomatoes, and onion and set aside.

In a small mixing bowl, combine the oil, vinegar, sugar, mustard, chopped chives, salt, and pepper and stir vigorously with a wire whisk. Allow the dressing to sit for at least 10 minutes to marry the flavors.

Pour the dressing over the salad and gently toss to ensure complete coverage. Transfer the salad to a serving bowl and garnish with the chive stems in the shape of an X against the rim of the bowl.

NUTRITIONAL ANALYSIS

EACH WITH: Calories: 73.75, Protein: 2.01 g, Carbs: 5.92 g, Total Fat: 5.17 g, Sat Fat: 0.73 g, Cholesterol: 0.03 mg, Sodium: 64.00 mg, Sugars: 3.66 g, Fiber: 1.44 g

Fresh Mediterranean Salad

TEXTURE: REGULAR

2 tablespoons (30 ml) red wine vinegar

2 tablespoons (30 ml) water

1 teaspoon dried oregano

1 teaspoon black pepper

1 teaspoon Dijon mustard

½ teaspoon kosher salt

2 cloves garlic, finely chopped

3 tablespoons (45 ml) extra-virgin olive oil

For Salad:

2 cups (174 g) sliced fennel bulb

1½ (240 g) cups thinly sliced red onion

1 cup (160 g) sliced black olives

¾ cup (45 g) fresh parsley, chopped

½ cup (75 g) crumbled feta cheese

1 can (15½ ounces, or 439 g) cannellini beans, rinsed and drained

6 plum tomatoes, quartered

—

Yield: Makes 12 (about ½-cup) servings

To make the vinaigrette: Combine the vinegar, water, oregano, pepper, mustard, salt, and garlic in a bowl. Slowly drizzle in the olive oil while whisking to blend.

To make the salad: Combine the fennel, red onion, olives, parsley, feta cheese, beans, and tomatoes in a large bowl. Toss the salad with the vinaigrette, cover, and chill for at least 1 hour before serving.

NUTRITIONAL ANALYSIS

EACH WITH: Calories: 111.94, Protein: 4.45 g, Carbs: 11.95 g, Total Fat: 5.54 g, Sat Fat: 1.16 g, Cholesterol: 1.67 mg, Sodium: 344.97 mg, Sugars: 2.48 g, Fiber: 3.55 g

Radicchio and Cauliflower Salad with Roasted Walnuts

TEXTURE: REGULAR

This colorful, festive salad is great for home entertaining or everyday enjoyment.

1 tablespoon (8 g) finely chopped walnuts

1 large radicchio head, quartered lengthwise, then sliced crosswise into thin strips

1 small cauliflower head, cut into small florets

½ small red onion, thinly sliced (about ⅓ cup, or 35 g)

½ cup (4 ounces, or 115 g) feta cheese

1 clove garlic, minced

1 tablespoon (14 ml) balsamic vinegar

1 teaspoon Dijon mustard

2 teaspoons minced shallot

1 teaspoon chopped fresh oregano

2 tablespoons (28 ml) olive oil

⅛ teaspoon salt

1 pinch freshly ground black pepper

—
Yield: Makes 6 (about ½-cup) servings

Preheat the oven to 375°F (190°C, or gas mark 5).

Place the walnuts on a sheet pan and bake for about 12 minutes, until the walnuts just begin to brown. Remove the sheet pan from the oven and set aside, allowing nuts to cool completely before adding them to the salad.

In a large bowl, mix the radicchio, cauliflower, and onion. Crumble the feta over the salad.

In a small bowl, whisk together the garlic, vinegar, mustard, shallot, and oregano. Slowly whisk in the oil. Season with the salt and pepper and mix the dressing into the salad. Let the salad sit for 1 hour in the refrigerator and top with toasted walnuts just prior to serving.

NUTRITIONAL ANALYSIS

EACH WITH: Calories: 109.52, Protein: 4.70 g, Carbs: 5.65 g, Total Fat: 8.35 g, Sat Fat: 3.29 g, Cholesterol: 16.68 mg, Sodium: 293.74 mg, Sugars: 3.09 g, Fiber: 1.55 g

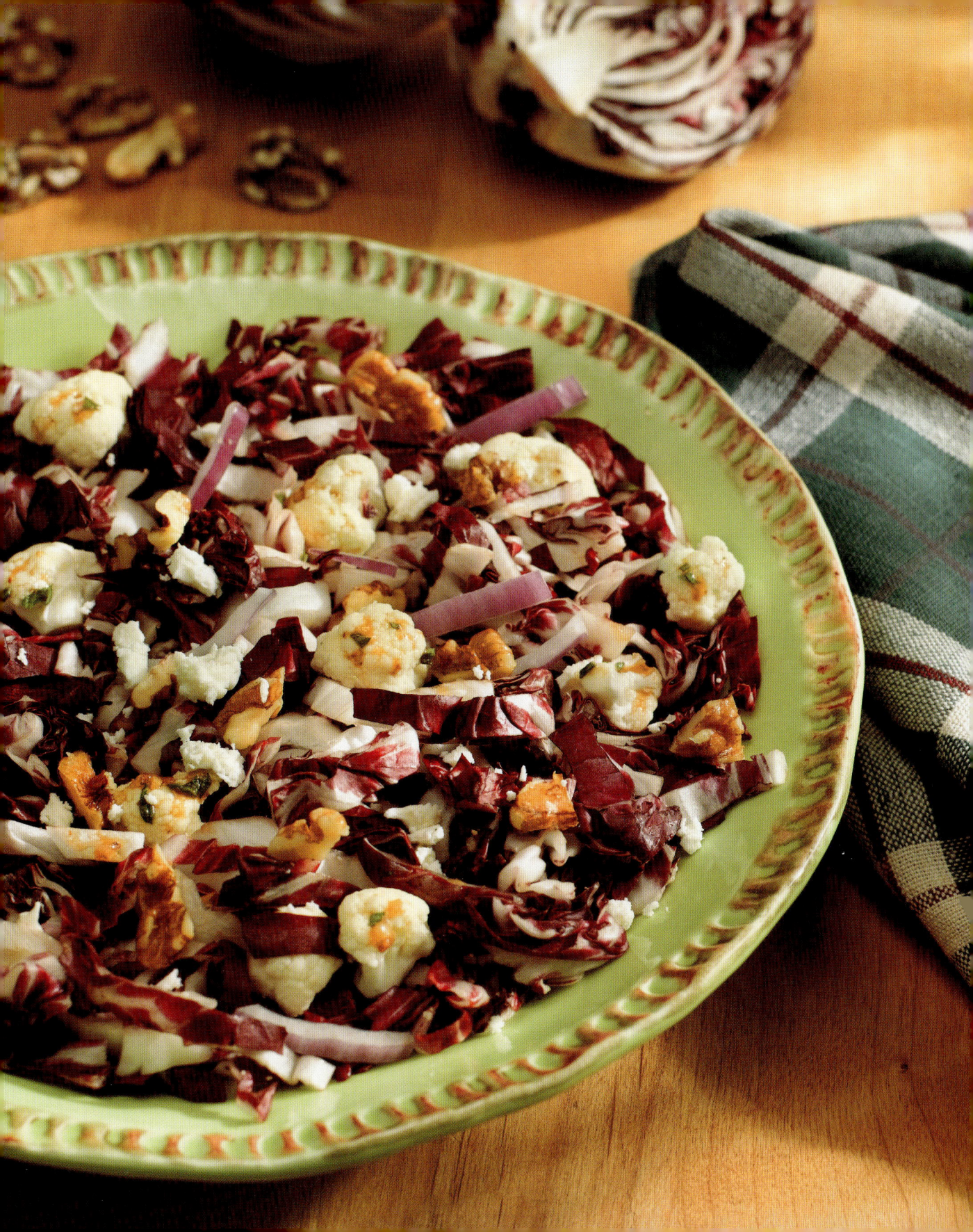

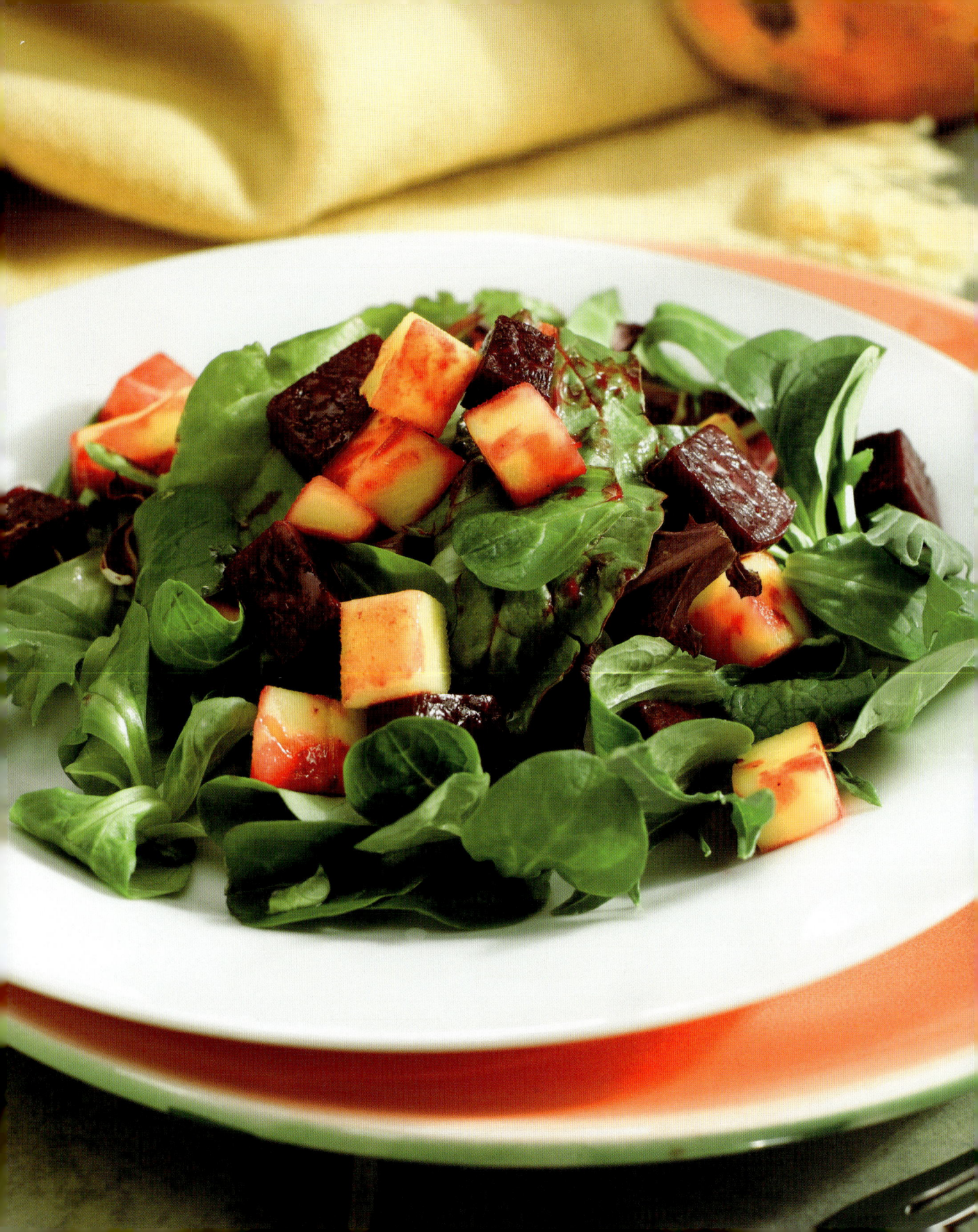

Roasted Beets and Mango Salad

2 medium beets, peeled and cut into 1-inch (2.5-cm) cubes (about ¾ pound, or 340 g)

¼ (60 ml) cup 100% orange juice

2 tablespoons (28 ml) fresh lime juice

½ teaspoon black pepper

1 tablespoon (15 g) Dijon mustard

2 teaspoons extra-virgin olive oil

⅛ teaspoon sea salt or kosher salt

1 cup (165 g) cubed ripe mango (about 2 mangoes)

6 cups (120 g) mixed field greens or gourmet salad mix

—

Yield: Makes 6 (about 1-cup) servings

Preheat the oven to 425°F (220°C, or gas mark 7).

In a 2-quart (2-L) saucepan, place the beets and cover with water to 1 inch (2.5 cm) above the level of the beets. Boil for 7 minutes, and then drain the beets in a colander.

Spray a 7½- x 11½-inch (17.5- x 27.5-cm) baking dish with cooking spray. Place the beats in the dish and roast for 30 minutes, until the beets are tender. Place beets in mixing bowl and cool in refrigerator.

In a 1 quart (1-L) mixing bowl, combine the orange juice, lime juice, pepper, mustard, oil, and salt. Mix vigorously with a wire whip or a fork and divide into two equal portions. Add one portion of the dressing to the beets and toss to cover all of the beet surface.

Remove the beets, reserving the remaining dressing. Combine the two portions of the remaining dressing.

In a large mixing bowl, place the salad greens. Pour the dressing over the salad greens. Gently toss to ensure complete exposure of the greens to the dressing.

Add the mangos to the beets and gently fold just enough to disperse beets and mangos evenly.

Divide the salad mixture among six chilled salad plates and top each salad with an equal amount of the beet-mango mixture.

NUTRITIONAL ANALYSIS

EACH WITH: Calories: 63.92, Protein: 1.52 g, Carbs: 11.88 g, Total Fat: 1.90 g, Sat Fat: 0.25 g, Cholesterol: 0.00 mg, Sodium: 98.43 mg, Sugars: 8.67 g, Fiber: 2.65 g,

Watercress Salad with Tarragon and Mint Leaves

TEXTURE: REGULAR

This is perfect as an accompaniment to Baked Sea Bass (page 121).

1 tablespoon (14 ml) olive oil

3 tablespoons (45 ml) apple cider vinegar

2 teaspoons lemon juice

¼ teaspoon salt

¼ teaspoon black pepper

2 cups (70 g) watercress

¼ cup (6 g) fresh spearmint leaves

¼ cup (15 g) fresh tarragon leaves

—

Yield: Makes 4 servings

In a small bowl, combine the oil, vinegar, and lemon juice and whisk briefly until emulsified. Add the salt and pepper.

In a serving bowl, place the watercress, mint, and tarragon. Pour the dressing on top and gently toss with salad tongs, just enough to ensure complete coverage.

NUTRITIONAL ANALYSIS

EACH WITH: Calories: 42.44, Protein: 1.03 g, Carbs: 4.96 g, Total Fat: 3.69 g, Sat Fat: 0.55 g, Cholesterol: 0.00 mg, Sodium: 98.07 mg, Sugars: 3.10 g, Fiber: 0.64 g

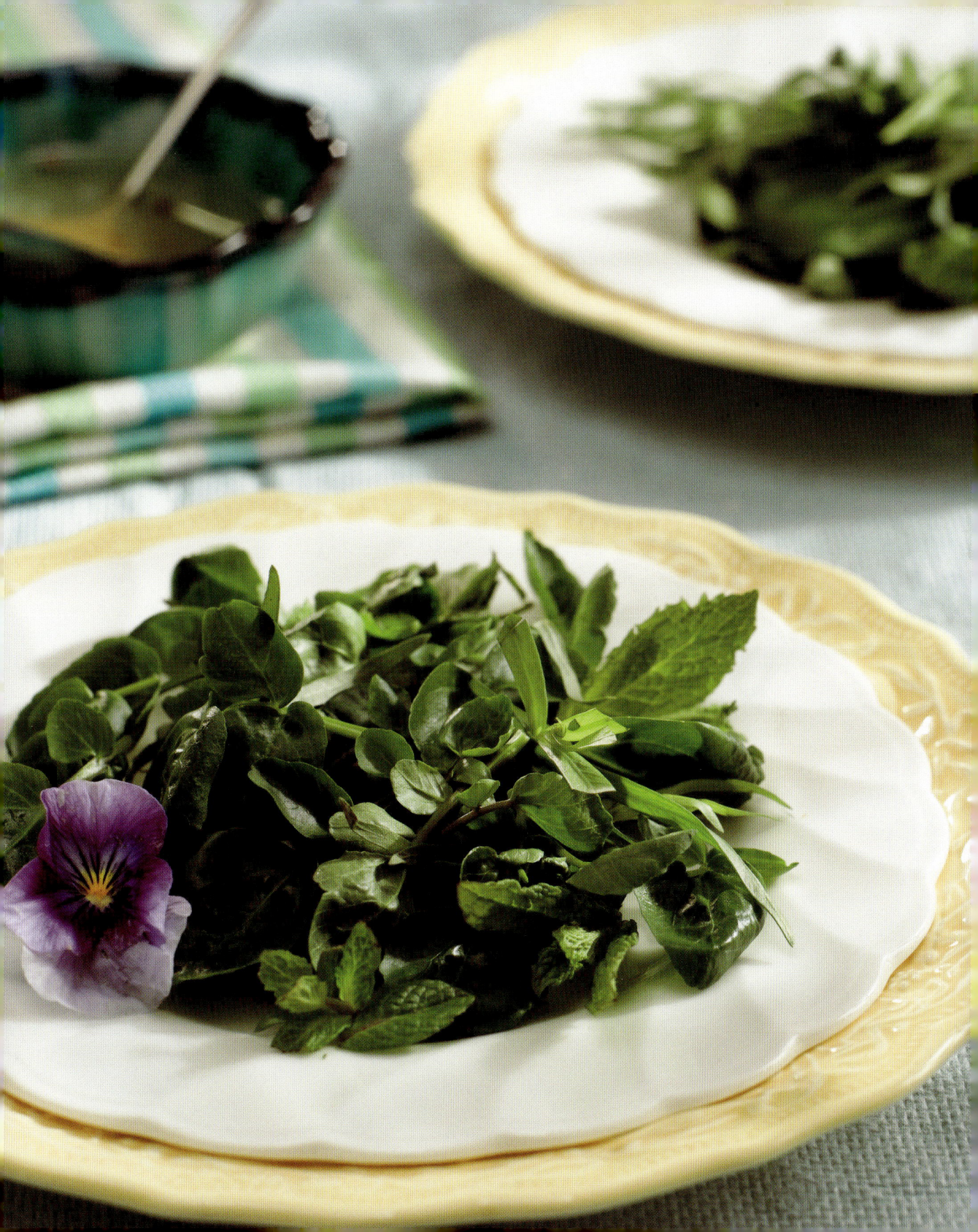

Creamy Lemon Herb Dressing

TEXTURE: PUREED

This low-fat (non-oil-based) salad dressing is the perfect alternative to the same old store-bought flavors. Making delicious salad dressing is really just this simple!

1 cup (225 g) nonfat cottage cheese

⅓ cup (75 ml) low-fat buttermilk

2 teaspoons fresh lemon juice

½ teaspoon lemon zest

1 teaspoon chopped fresh tarragon leaves

1 teaspoon chopped fresh parsley

1 teaspoon chopped fresh green onion (white and green parts)

—

Yield: Makes 10 (about 2-tablespoon) servings

Place all of the ingredients in a blender or food processor and blend until smooth.

NUTRITIONAL ANALYSIS

EACH WITH: Calories: 19.84, Protein: 2.90 g, Carbs: 1.74 g, Total Fat: 0.08 g, Sat Fat: 0.05 g, Cholesterol: 1.33 mg, Sodium: 96.71 mg, Sugars: 1.42 g, Fiber: 0.03 g

Blue Cheese Dressing

TEXTURE: PUREED

1 cup (225 g) nonfat cottage cheese

⅓ cup (75 ml) nonfat buttermilk

2 tablespoons (15 g) blue cheese crumbles

½ teaspoon Worcestershire sauce

½ teaspoon fresh lemon juice

1 teaspoon finely chopped fresh parsley

½ teaspoon black pepper

—

Yield: Makes 10 (about 2-tablespoon) servings

Place all of the ingredients in a blender or food processor and blend until smooth.

NUTRITIONAL ANALYSIS

EACH WITH: Calories: 24.88, Protein: 3.23 g, Carbs: 1.76 g, Total Fat: 0.51 g, Sat Fat: 0.29 g, Cholesterol: 2.33 mg, Sodium: 115.72 mg, Sugars: 1.43 g, Fiber: 0.03 g

Sweet Lemon Poppy Seed Dressing

TEXTURE: PUREED

1 cup (225 g) nonfat cottage cheese

⅓ cup (75 ml) low-fat buttermilk

2 teaspoons fresh lemon juice

½ teaspoon lemon zest

2 teaspoons honey

1 teaspoon poppy seeds

Place all of the ingredients in a blender or food processor and blend until smooth.

—

Yield: Makes 10 (about 2-tablespoon) servings

NUTRITIONAL ANALYSIS

EACH WITH: Calories: 25.06, Protein: 2.93 g, Carbs: 2.83 g, Total Fat: 0.20 g, Sat Fat: 0.06 g, Cholesterol: 1.33 mg, Sodium: 96.65 mg, Sugars: 2.52 g, Fiber: 0.04 g

Garden Goddess Dressing

TEXTURE: PUREED

1 cup (225 g) nonfat cottage cheese

⅓ cup (75 ml) low-fat buttermilk

1 teaspoon fresh lemon juice

2 teaspoons anchovy paste

1 tablespoon (4 g) chopped fresh parsley

2 teaspoons chopped green onion

1 teaspoon chopped fresh oregano leaves (stems removed)

Place all of the ingredients in a blender or food processor and blend until smooth.

—

Yield: Makes 10 (about 2-tablespoon) servings

NUTRITIONAL ANALYSIS

EACH WITH: Calories: 21.94, Protein: 3.04 g, Carbs: 1.75 g, Total Fat: 0.25 g, Sat Fat: 0.08 g, Cholesterol: 4.99 mg, Sodium: 159.49 mg, Sugars: 1.42 g, Fiber: 0.07 g

CHAPTER 4

Appetizers and Entertaining at Home

Vegetable Party Platter

TEXTURE: REGULAR

Serve with the delicious Smoked Salmon Dip (page 90) for a festive dish.

8 whole leaves red leaf lettuce

1 red bell pepper, cut into strips

1 yellow bell pepper, cut into strips

3 Italian plum tomatoes, cored and cut into 4 wedges each

½ cauliflower head, cut into bite-size florets

—

Yield: Makes 12 (about ¼-cup) servings

On a large serving platter, spread out the lettuce leaves. Arrange the vegetable pieces around the outside of the bowl.

NUTRITIONAL ANALYSIS

EACH WITH: Calories: 25.66, Protein: 1.30 g, Carbs: 5.46 g, Total Fat: 0.23 g, Sat Fat: 0.04 g, Cholesterol: 0.00 mg, Sodium: 12.80 mg, Sugars: 3.43 g, Fiber: 1.95 g

Sweet Corn Relish

TEXTURE: MECHANICAL SOFT

Try this zesty relish as a topping for fish or chicken or for a dip with Toasted Pita Chips (page 86).

1½ cups (240 g) fresh corn kernels (about 4 large ears, shucked)

½ medium red bell pepper, cored and finely chopped (about ½ cup, or 70 g)

2 tablespoons (20 g) finely chopped red onion

1 teaspoon finely chopped fresh jalapeno pepper, seeds removed

2 teaspoons chopped fresh cilantro

1 small clove garlic, minced

1 teaspoon salt

¼ teaspoon black pepper

—

Yield: Makes 8 (about ¼-cup) servings

In a small bowl, combine all ingredients and stir to mix. Cover and refrigerate for 30 minutes, stirring once or twice before serving.

NUTRITIONAL ANALYSIS

EACH WITH: Calories: 38.95, Protein: 1.25 g, Carbs: 8.86 g, Total Fat: 0.43 g, Sat Fat: 0.06 g, Cholesterol: 0.00 mg, Sodium: 42.17 mg, Sugars: 1.87 g, Fiber: 1.24 g

Curry Yogurt Dip

TEXTURE: PUREED

Serve with Toasted Pita Chips (page 86) and fresh vegetable sticks. It can be made up to 24 hours ahead of time.

1 cup (225 g) nonfat cottage cheese

3 tablespoons (45 g) nonfat mayonnaise

1 green onion, thinly sliced (white and green parts)

3 teaspoons chopped fresh cilantro

1½ teaspoons curry powder

⅛ teaspoon cayenne pepper (optional)

—
Yield: Makes 8 (about 2-tablespoons) servings

In a food processor, blend the cottage cheese for about 30 seconds, until smooth.

Using a rubber spatula, scrape the cottage cheese into a small mixing bowl and add the mayonnaise, onion, cilantro, curry powder, and cayenne pepper (if using). Stir to combine, place in a serving bowl, cover, and refrigerate until ready to serve.

NUTRITIONAL ANALYSIS

EACH WITH: Calories: 25.43, Protein: 3.33 g, Carbs: 2.57 g, Total Fat: 0.06 g, Sat Fat: 0.01 g, Cholesterol: 1.25 mg, Sodium: 155.32 mg, Sugars: 1.67 g, Fiber: 0.19 g

Tzatziki

TEXTURE: MECHANICAL SOFT

This is a delicious Greek-style cool and creamy cucumber sauce that will freshen up just about any dish.

2 tablespoons (30 ml) extra-virgin olive oil

1 tablespoon (15 ml) white wine vinegar

2 cloves garlic, finely minced

½ teaspoon kosher salt

¼ teaspoon white pepper

1 cup (230 g) plain, low-fat Greek yogurt

1 cup (230 g) fat-free sour cream

2 medium cucumbers, peeled, seeded, and finely chopped

1 teaspoon fresh dill, chopped

—
Yield: Makes about 30 (about ¼-cup) servings

Combine the olive oil, vinegar, garlic, salt, and pepper in a bowl. Mix well.

Strain the yogurt through a coffee filter set in a strainer in the refrigerator for 2 to 3 hours. After the yogurt has strained, blend it, using a whisk, with the sour cream until smooth.

Next, combine the olive oil mixture with the yogurt mixture. Add the cucumber and dill. Chill for at least 2 hours before serving.

NUTRITIONAL ANALYSIS

EACH WITH: Calories: 24.56, Protein: 1.25 g, Carbs: 2.27 g, Total Fat: 1.20 g, Sat Fat: 0.30 g, Cholesterol: 1.27 mg, Sodium: 40.68 mg, Sugars: 1.32 g, Fiber: 0.21 g

Fresh Salsa Caliente

TEXTURE: SOFT

1 cup (180 g) coarsely chopped tomato

¼ cup (40 g) coarsely chopped yellow
or red onion

1 small jalapeno pepper, finely chopped
(optional)

2 tablespoons (2 g) chopped fresh cilantro

¼ teaspoon salt

¼ teaspoon cracked black pepper

—

Yield: Makes 6 (about ¼-cup) servings

Place the tomato, onion, and jalapeno pepper
(if using) in a food processor fitted with a metal
blade. Pulse the mixture just enough to break the
pieces down to a bit smaller size. Add the cilantro,
salt, and pepper and pulse one or two more times.

NUTRITIONAL ANALYSIS

EACH WITH: Calories: 11.98, Protein: 0.47 g,
Carbs: 2.62 g, Total Fat: 0.16 g, Sat Fat: 0.02 g,
Cholesterol: 0.00 mg, Sodium: 71.84 mg,
Sugars: 1.39 g, Fiber: 0.64 g

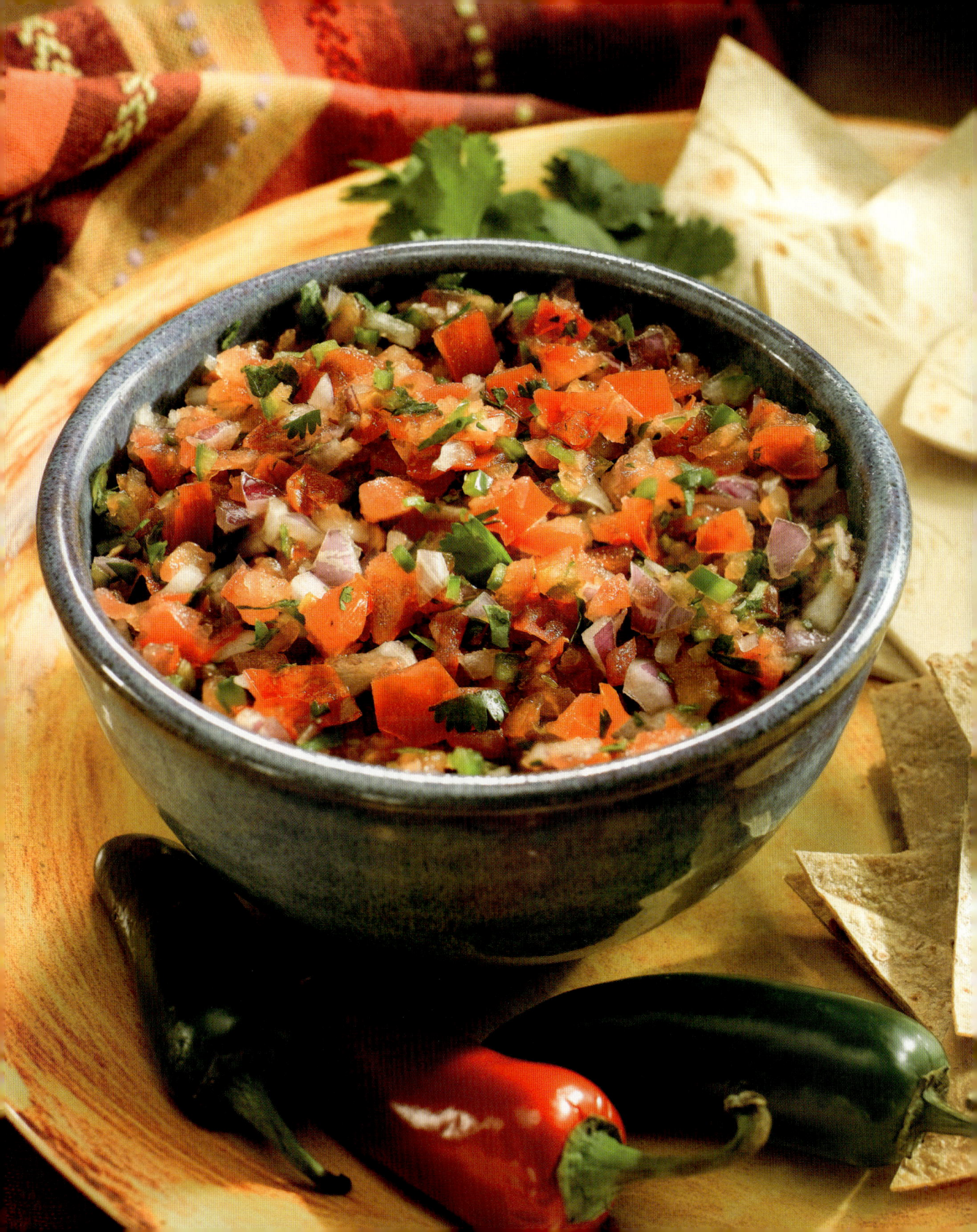

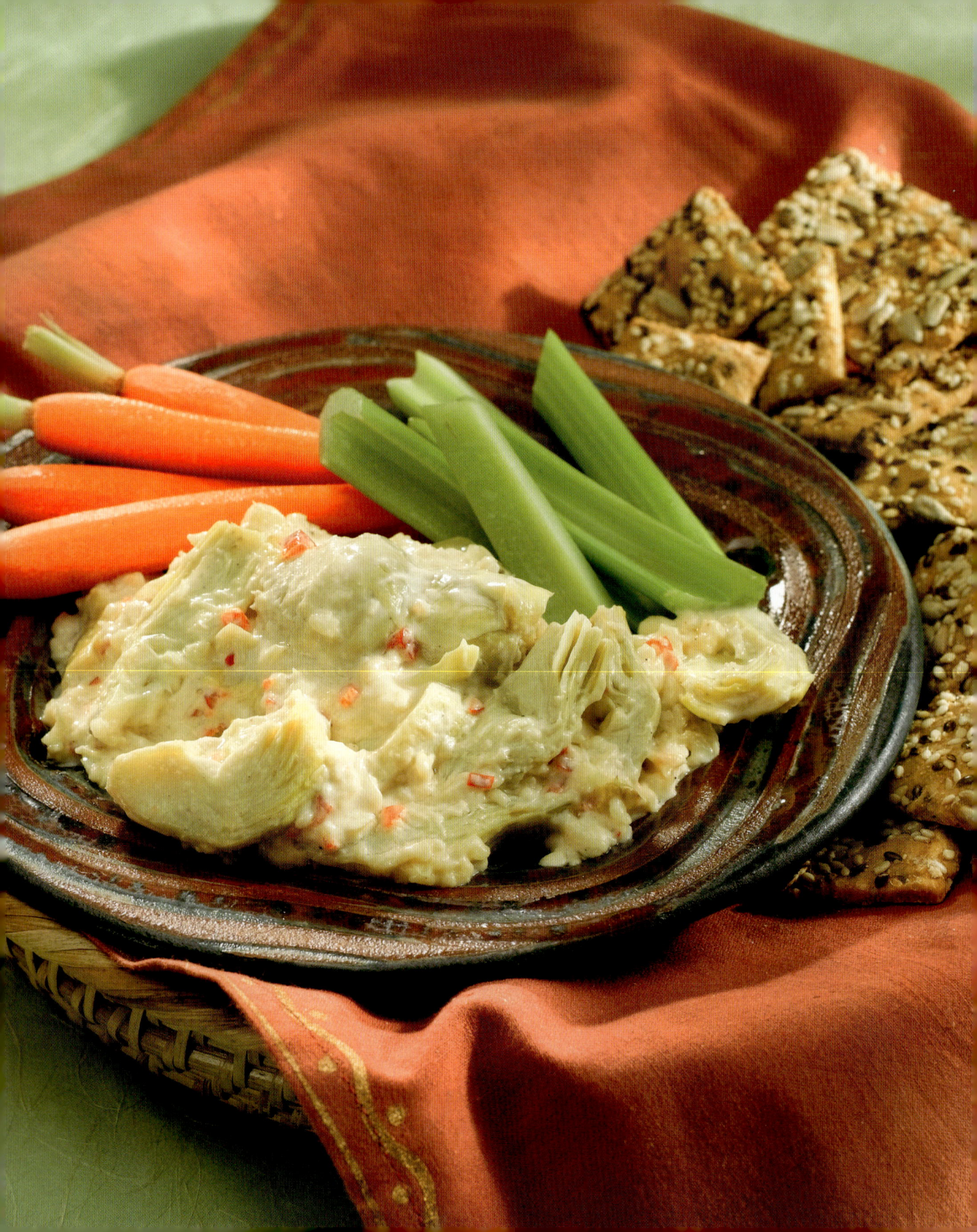

Hot Artichoke Dip

TEXTURE: SOFT (RAW VEGETABLES AS PICTURED: REGULAR)

This is a simple, healthy, delicious dip that will get your party started right. I make it for parties, and it's always a hit! For added color and a little more flavor, add 1 tablespoon (10 g) finely chopped red pepper. For a little extra kick, add 1 finely chopped small fresh jalapeno pepper. For more fiber, serve with low-fat, whole wheat crackers.

2 cans (14 ounces, 400 g each) artichoke hearts, drained and cut into quarters

1 cup (110 g) shredded low-moisture, part-skim mozzarella cheese

¾ cup (175 g) nonfat mayonnaise

¼ cup (20 g) shredded Parmesan cheese

⅛ teaspoon salt

¼ teaspoon black pepper

—

Yield: Makes 10 (about ½-cup) servings

Preheat the oven to 375°F (190°C, or gas mark 5).

In a 1-quart (1-L) casserole oven-safe dish, place the artichoke hearts. Add the mozzarella cheese, mayonnaise, Parmesan cheese, salt, and pepper. Mix thoroughly with a large spoon, ensuring even distribution. Bake the dip for 15 minutes and serve immediately. (Avoid overheating to ensure the mayonnaise does not separate.)

NUTRITIONAL ANALYSIS

EACH WITH: Calories: 74.47, Protein: 4.97 g, Carbs: 7.30 g, Total Fat: 2.35 g, Sat Fat: 1.55 g, Cholesterol: 7.44 mg, Sodium: 456.30 mg, Sugars: 1.87 g, Fiber: 1.21 g

Toasted Pita Chips

TEXTURE: REGULAR

Pita chips are a great alternative to high-fat corn or potato chips and can be flavored in a variety of ways. This recipe is plain and simple to complement the scrumptious flavor of Roasted Garlic at right.

1 tablespoon (14 ml) olive oil

6 (6-inch, or 15 cm) whole-wheat pita breads (see note)

½ teaspoon celery salt

½ teaspoon paprika

⅛ teaspoon black pepper

—

Yield: Makes 48 chips; 1 serving is about 4 pita chips.

Preheat the oven to 375°F (190°C, or gas mark 5). Using a pastry brush, lightly brush oil onto both sides of each pita. Cut the pitas into 8 wedges each. In a small bowl, combine the celery salt, paprika, and pepper. Place the pitas on a baking sheet and sprinkle one side with the seasoning mixture. Bake the pitas for about 15 minutes, until the chips are beginning to turn golden brown.

MARGARET'S NOTE

You could use low-carb whole-wheat pita bread instead of regular whole-wheat pita to lower the calories and increase the protein of the pita chips.

Roasted Garlic

TEXTURE: PUREE

Roasted garlic is versatile and easy to prepare. (It's also easy on the breath after it's cooked!) In addition to the Toasted Pita Chips (left), try spreading some on a toasted English muffin with scrambled egg substitute for breakfast.

10 garlic bulbs

Olive oil

—

Yield: 12 servings

Preheat the oven to 300°F (150°C, or gas mark 2). Peel away the papery skin on the outside of the garlic bulbs, but leave the cloves attached. Rub some olive oil on your hands, then rub the whole bulbs of garlic just enough to give them a slightly shiny appearance. Wrap the bulbs in aluminum foil and place on a sheet pan. Roast the garlic for 1 hour, until the cloves are soft. (You will surely smell it cooking before it's done!) Unwrap the garlic and allow it to cool to the touch before squeezing out the soft, delicious pulp.

NUTRITIONAL ANALYSIS

EACH WITH: Calories: 100.00, Protein: 3.31 g, Carbs: 18.49 g, Total Fat: 2.02 g, Sat Fat: 0.30 g, Cholesterol: 0.00 mg, Sodium: 218.61 mg, Sugars: 0.30 g, Fiber: 2.46 g

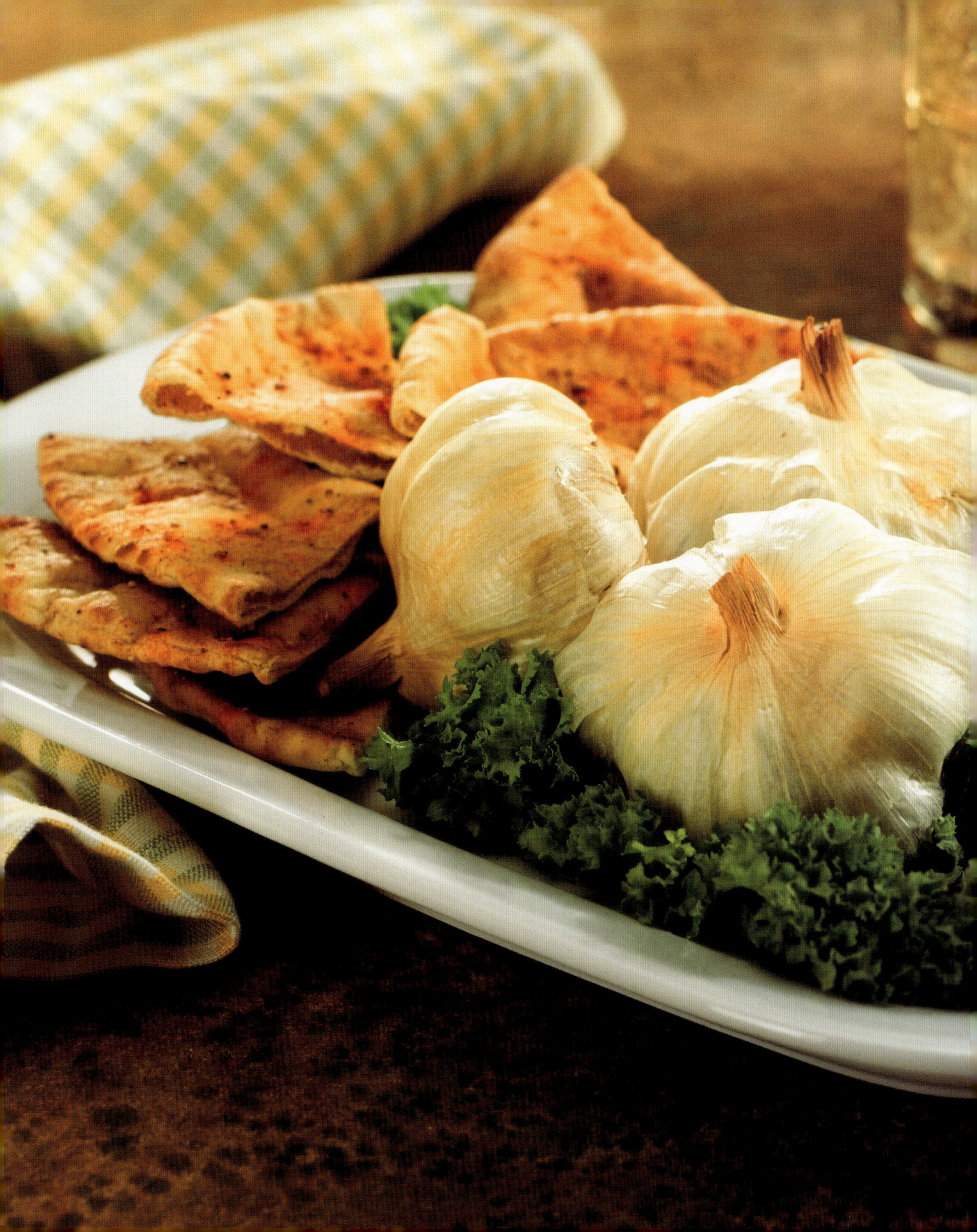

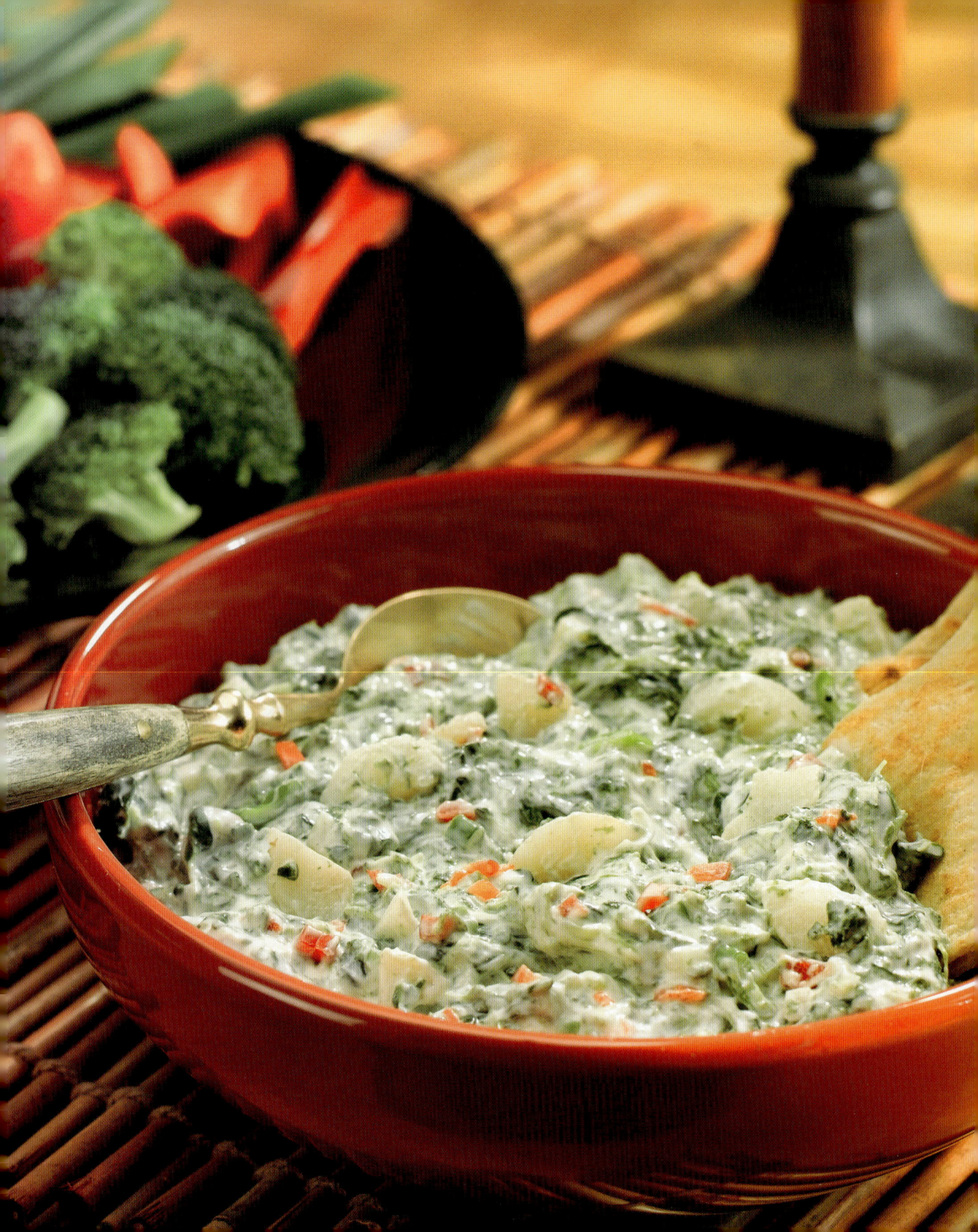

Easy and Delicious Spinach Dip

TEXTURE: SOFT

This dip is great with fresh vegetable sticks or whole wheat pita—a party favorite!

1 package (10 ounces, or 280 g) frozen, chopped spinach

½ cup (50 g) chopped green onion

¼ teaspoon garlic powder

2 tablespoons (20 g) finely chopped red bell pepper

¼ cup (50 g) water chestnuts, drained and chopped

1 cup (200 g) nonfat sour cream

1 cup (230 g) nonfat mayonnaise

1 tablespoon (14 ml) lemon juice

½ teaspoon salt

¼ teaspoon black pepper, ground

—
Yield: Makes 14 (about ¼-cup) servings

Thaw and drain the spinach in a colander, pressing all of the excess moisture out.

In a medium mixing bowl, mix the onion, garlic powder, bell pepper, water chestnuts, sour cream, mayonnaise, lemon juice, salt, and black pepper until well incorporated.

NUTRITIONAL ANALYSIS

EACH WITH: Calories: 41.66, Protein: 1.85 g, Carbs: 7.78 g, Total Fat: 0.10 g, Sat Fat: 0.01 g, Cholesterol: 2.86 mg, Sodium: 250.37 mg, Sugars: 2.82 g, Fiber: 0.79 g

Smoked Salmon Dip

TEXTURE: SOFT

Smoked salmon is always a hit at parties. This dip has tangy kick to it.

1 cup (225 g) nonfat cottage cheese

½ cup (100 g) nonfat sour cream

¾ cup (6 ounces, or 170 g) chopped smoked salmon

3 large green onions, thinly sliced (white and green parts)

2 teaspoons fresh lemon juice

⅛ teaspoon cayenne pepper (optional)

—

Yield: Makes about 10 (2-tablespoons) servings

In a food processor, blend the cottage cheese for about 30 seconds, until smooth. Using a rubber spatula, scrape the cottage cheese into a medium mixing bowl. Add the sour cream, salmon, onions, lemon juice, and cayenne pepper (if using). Mix well. Place the dip into a serving bowl and refrigerate until ready to serve.

NUTRITIONAL ANALYSIS

EACH WITH: Calories: 54.70, Protein: 7.04 g, Carbs: 3.79 g, Total Fat: 1.20 g, Sat Fat: 0.40 g, Cholesterol: 10.00 mg, Sodium: 312.08 mg, Sugars: 1.86 g, Fiber: 0.07 g

Latkes

This is a great dish for parties.

3 pounds (1.5 kg) Yukon gold potatoes, skinned and finely grated (see note)

1 cup (160 g) finely diced yellow onion

¾ cup (85 g) finely grated carrot

½ cup (50 g) finely chopped green onion

½ cup (30 g) finely chopped parsley

⅓ cup (45 g) matzo meal

½ teaspoon baking powder

1 cup (235 ml) liquid egg substitute or egg whites

1 teaspoon kosher salt

¼ teaspoon black pepper

2 teaspoons granulated garlic

½ cup (50 g) grated Parmesan cheese

⅓ cup (75 ml) olive oil

—
Yield: Makes 50 to 60 (2-inch) latkes, which should serve about 15 people.

Heat a heavy baking sheet or a large cast-iron skillet in the oven at 450°F (230°C, or gas mark 8).

Drain the potatoes, yellow onion, carrot, green onion, and parsley by pressing them into a fine mesh strainer or by squeezing them in cheese-cloth. Once all excess moisture is removed, transfer the grated vegetables to a large (at least 3 quart, or 3-L) mixing bowl. Add the matzo meal, baking powder, egg substitute or egg whites, salt, pepper, garlic, and cheese and mix to incorporate well.

Remove the baking sheet or skillet from the oven. Using a pastry brush, lightly brush it with the oil. Immediately spoon ¼ cup (60 ml) of the latke batter onto the sheet or skillet and return the pan to the oven. Bake for 7 to 10 minutes on each side, until a golden brown color appears. This can be done in batches, making several at a time. Remember to heat the baking sheet then brush it with olive oil just prior to cooking each batch.

NOTE
You can grate the potatoes by hand or in a food processor fitted with a fine grating disc.

NUTRITIONAL ANALYSIS:

2-latkes with: Calories: 139.85, Protein: 6.17 g, Carbs: 21.87 g, Total Fat: 3.42 g, Sat Fat: 1.16 g, Cholesterol: 1.77 mg, Sodium: 246.62 mg, Sugars: 2.36 g, Fiber: 2.87 g

Pacific Dungeness Crab Cakes

TEXTURE: SOFT

These crab cakes contain no bread or flour fillers, just pure, delicious Dungeness crab!

½ pound (225 g) Dungeness crabmeat, cooked (any cooked crabmeat may be substituted, except for canned)

1 tablespoon (16 g) minced celery

2 teaspoons minced red bell pepper

2 teaspoons finely chopped fresh cilantro

2 tablespoons (30 g) nonfat mayonnaise

⅛ teaspoon sea salt or kosher salt

⅛ teaspoon cayenne pepper (optional)

2 teaspoons olive oil

½ teaspoon toasted sesame oil

2 tablespoons (2 g) gourmet salad greens

2 lemon wedges

2 tablespoons (30 g) low-fat tartar sauce

—

Yield: Makes 6 (about 1½ -ounces) crab cakes

Place the crabmeat in a strainer or colander and press out excess moisture.

Transfer the crabmeat to a medium mixing bowl, and add the celery, bell pepper, and cilantro.

In a small bowl, combine the mayonnaise, salt, and cayenne pepper (if using) and stir to mix.

Add the mayonnaise mixture to the crabmeat and mix until well incorporated.

Form the mixture into 6 equal patties (about 2 ounces, or 55 g each), pressing firmly enough to hold together, and place on waxed paper on top of a plate. Cover the top of the crab cakes with another sheet of waxed paper and refrigerate for 15 minutes.

In a medium, nonstick skillet, heat the olive oil and sesame oil over medium-high heat and swirl the pan to mix the oils. Gently place the crab cakes in the pan using a thin metal spatula and cook undisturbed for about 6 minutes on each side, until well browned, manipulating them only to avoid burning, then remove the pan from heat.

Place 1 tablespoon (1 g) of the greens in a pile on the center of a plate and place the crab cakes on the pile, leaning off of one side. Place a lemon wedge beside the greens and crab cakes and a teaspoon of the tartar sauce atop each cake.

NUTRITIONAL ANALYSIS

EACH WITH: Calories: 70.57, Protein: 8.49 g, Carbs: 2.43 g, Total Fat: 2.68 g, Sat Fat: 0.29 g, Cholesterol: 28.73 mg, Sodium: 269.31 mg, Sugars: 1.32 g, Fiber: 0.12 g

NOTE

Two crab cakes equal the portion recommendation for an entrée serving, or one crab cake can be served as an appetizer. A little goes a long way with crabmeat, as it has a very rich flavor and texture.

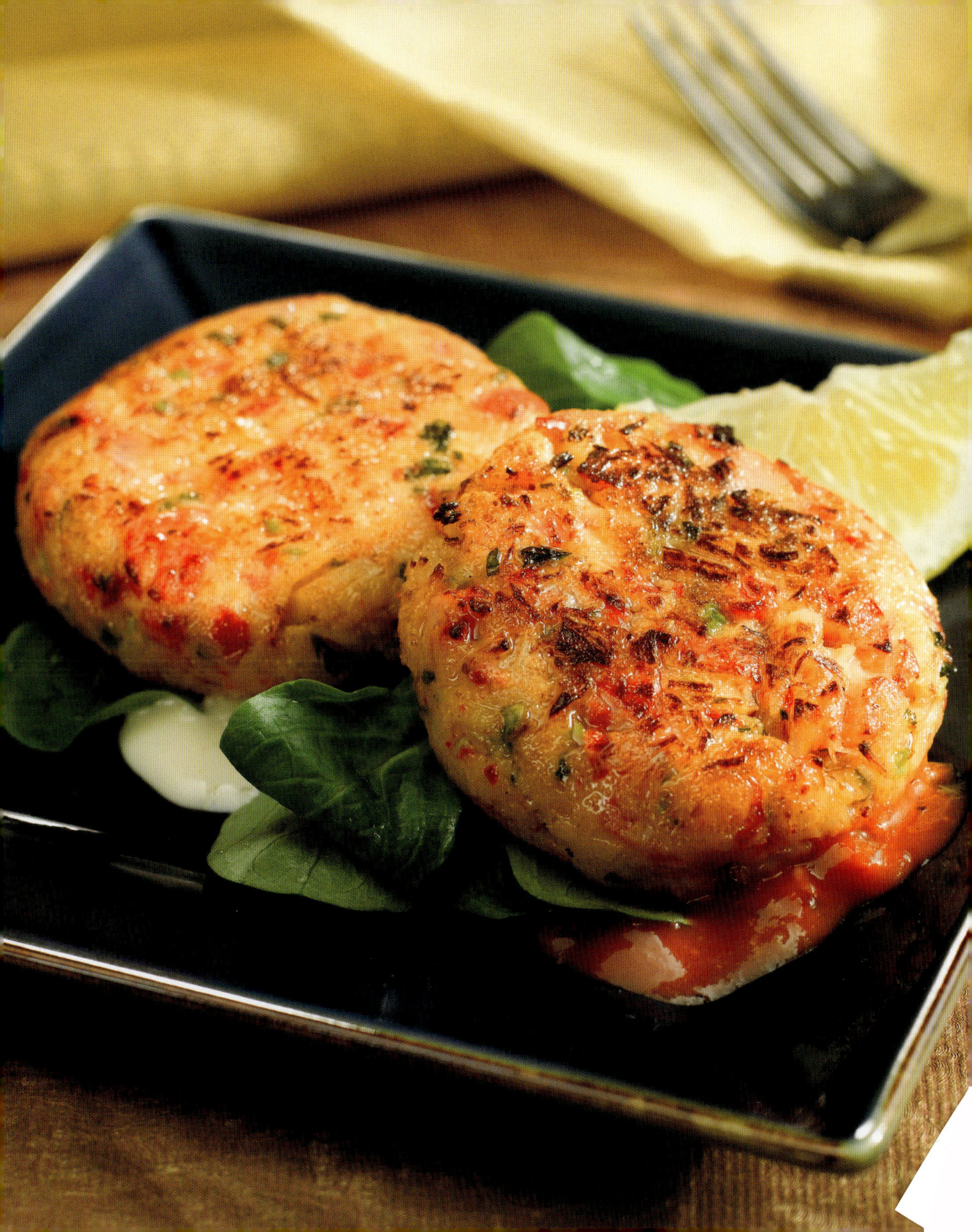

BBQ Turkey Meatballs

TEXTURE: SOFT

This recipe calls for brown sugar substitute; choose one that's suitable in cooking applications (see page 18).

1 pound (450 g) ground turkey

1 cup (160 g) chopped onion

3 tablespoons (45 g) liquid egg substitute

¼ cup (60 ml) low-fat milk

¼ cup (30 g) whole-wheat bread crumbs

1 teaspoon kosher salt

¼ teaspoon black pepper

2 tablespoons (28 ml) extra-virgin olive oil

2 cans (8 ounces, or 360 g each) tomato sauce

¼ cup (6 g) brown sugar substitute

2 tablespoons (28 ml) vinegar

1 teaspoon garlic powder

—

Yield: Makes 12 (about 4-ounce) meatballs

Combine the turkey, onion, egg substitute, milk, bread crumbs, salt, and pepper in a bowl. Mix thoroughly and shape into 12 meatballs.

Heat the olive oil in a large skillet over medium-high heat, and then brown the meatballs.

In a medium-size bowl, combine the tomato sauce, brown sugar substitute, vinegar, and garlic powder. Pour over the meatballs. Simmer over low heat for 10 to 15 minutes, turning frequently, until the meatballs are well glazed and are cooked through.

NUTRITIONAL ANALYSIS

EACH WITH: Calories: 120.96, Protein: 8.76 g, Carbs: 10.02 g, Total Fat: 5.73 g, Sat Fat: 1.19 g, Cholesterol: 29.96 mg, Sodium: 363.20 mg, Sugars: 4.79 g, Fiber: 1.86 g

JOE'S TIP

This would also be a great and easy slow cooker recipe that you could bring along to a party. Follow the recipe as it is written, but instead of simmering over low heat for 10 to 15 minutes, pour all the ingredients into the slow cooker and cook on the low setting for 4 to 6 hours, or until the meatballs are cooked through and tender.

Stuffed Mushrooms

TEXTURE: SOFT

This is another can't miss party favorite or dinner party appetizer and a great source of potassium.

1 pound (455 g) medium mushrooms (about 18)

1 tablespoon (14 ml) olive oil

1 clove garlic, minced

6 teaspoons finely diced red bell pepper

¼ cup (40 g) finely diced yellow onion

2 tablespoons (15 g) thinly sliced green onion (green and white parts)

1 tablespoon (4 g) chopped fresh parsley

¼ teaspoon dried basil

¼ teaspoon dried oregano

¾ cup (75 g) whole-wheat bread crumbs (about 1½ slices bread, toasted)

2 tablespoons (10 g) grated Parmesan cheese

—

Yield: Makes 6 (about ½-cup) servings

Preheat the oven to 375°F (190°C, or gas mark 5).

Clean the mushrooms and remove the stems. Finely chop or mince the stems and set aside.

Place the mushroom caps in a 9- x 13-inch (22.5- x 32.5-cm) baking dish.

In a medium nonstick skillet, heat the oil over medium-high heat. Add the mushroom stems and garlic and sauté for about 3 minutes. Add the bell pepper, yellow onion, green onion, parsley, basil, and oregano and continue cooking for about 4 minutes, until the peppers are soft. Remove from heat and add the bread crumbs and cheese. Stir to combine. Fill the mushroom caps with the stuffing mixture and bake for 20 minutes, until the mushrooms are soft.

NUTRITIONAL ANALYSIS

EACH WITH: Calories: 75.68, Protein: 4.14 g, Carbs: 7.26 g, Total Fat: 3.63 g, Sat Fat: 0.87 g, Cholesterol: 1.00 mg, Sodium: 81.86 mg, Sugars: 2.50 g, Fiber: 1.59 g

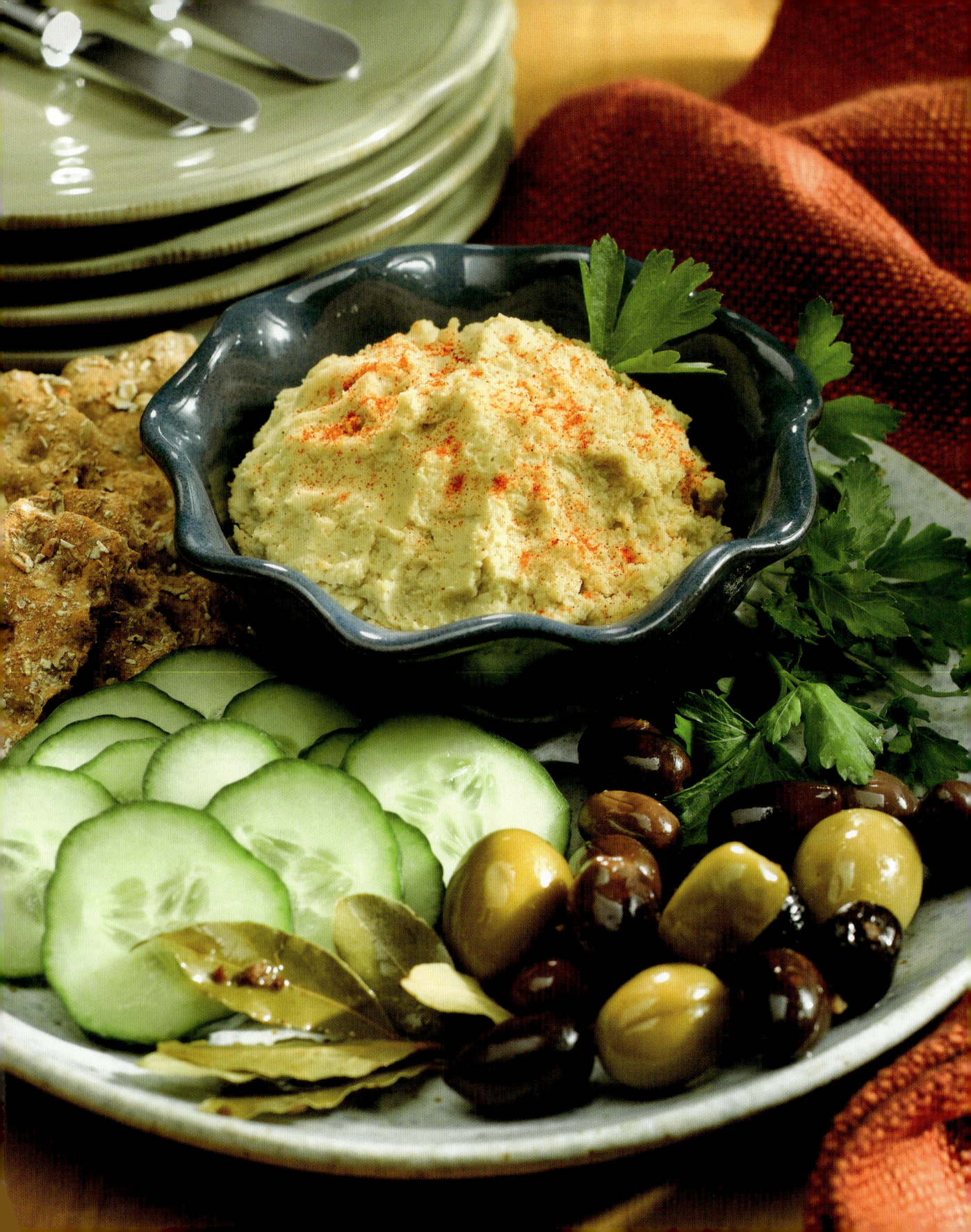

Traditional Hummus

Serve this with cucumber slices, tomato wedges, Greek olives, and pita bread. Note that five Greek olives equals one serving of fat.

3–5 cloves fresh garlic, crushed

1½ tablespoons (21 ml) extra-virgin olive oil, divided

3 cans (15 ounces, or 430 g each) cooked chickpeas (garbanzo beans), rinsed and drained

¼ cup (60 g) sesame tahini

½ teaspoon toasted sesame oil

2 tablespoons (28 ml) cold water

2 tablespoons (28 ml) fresh lemon juice

½ teaspoon salt

2 teaspoons ground cumin

—

Yield: Makes 16 (about ¼-cup) servings

Place the garlic in a food processor with 1½ teaspoons of the olive oil and process until the garlic is minced, almost paste-like. (You will need to stop the process and scrape down the garlic from the sides of the container a few times.) Add the chickpeas, tahini, sesame oil, water, lemon juice, salt, and cumin, and continue processing. While the puree is still processing, slowly add the remaining olive oil. (The consistency should have a smooth but grainy texture. If a thinner consistency is preferred, add additional water in small increments.)

NUTRITIONAL ANALYSIS:

EACH WITH: Calories: 111.99, Protein: 4.74 g, Carbs: 13.54 g, Total Fat: 4.68 g, Sat Fat: 0.59 g, Cholesterol: 0.00 mg, Sodium: 39.90 mg, Sugars: 2.35 g, Fiber: 3.89 g

Teresa's Edamame Dip

TEXTURE: PUREE

This dip, using super-healthy green soybeans, comes from Teresa, a gastric bypass surgery patient in Baltimore. You can find shelled edamame in the natural foods freezer section of most grocery stores.

2 cups (512 g) shelled edamame

1 cup (235 ml) water

½ teaspoon kosher salt, divided

2 cloves garlic, finely chopped

1 teaspoon lemon or lime zest

2 teaspoons lemon or lime juice

2 cups (460 g) plain nonfat yogurt

1 small cucumber, seeded, peeled, and chopped

1 cup (180 g) seeded and diced tomato

¼ cup (20 g) chopped turkey bacon, cooked

¼ cup (30 g) low-fat shredded Cheddar cheese

—

Yield: Makes 16 (about ¼-cup) servings

Bring the edamame, water, ¼ teaspoon salt, and garlic to a simmer for 15 to 20 minutes. Drain, reserving ¼ cup (59 ml) of the cooking liquid. Process the edamame until smooth in a food processor or blender. Add the lemon or lime zest and lemon or lime juice and blend. Set aside.

Strain the yogurt through a coffee filter set in a strainer in the refrigerator for 2 to 3 hours. After the yogurt has strained, mix it with the cucumber and remaining ¼ teaspoon salt.

Spread the edamame mixture on the bottom of a serving plate. Spoon the yogurt mixture over the top, and sprinkle with the tomatoes, turkey bacon, and Cheddar cheese.

NUTRITIONAL ANALYSIS

EACH WITH: Calories: 40.92, Protein: 3.92 g, Carbs: 4.71 g, Total Fat: 1.10 g, Sat Fat: 0.11 g, Cholesterol: 2.19 mg, Sodium: 126.27 mg, Sugars: 2.60 g, Fiber: 0.91 g

Protein-Packed 7-Layer Bean Dip

TEXTURE: REGULAR

This is a classic dish for entertaining that is always a big hit. It's also quick and easy to prepare.

2 cups (476 g) refried beans

1 teaspoon chipotle chili powder

½ teaspoon ground cumin

1 cup (115 g) shredded low-fat Cheddar cheese

¼ cup (30 g) chopped chile peppers,
or canned jalapeños

1 avocado, peeled and chopped

1 hot-house tomato, seeded and chopped

⅓ cup (77 g) fat-free sour cream

¼ cup (25 g) sliced black olives

2 scallions, sliced

—

Yield: Makes 8 (about ½-cup) servings

Heat the refried beans in a medium sauté pan over low heat. Stir in enough water to make them creamy. Mix in the chipotle chili powder and cumin.

Once the beans are hot, spread them over the bottom of a warmed serving dish. Immediately add the shredded Cheddar cheese. Layer on the chopped chile peppers (or jalapeños), avocado, tomato, and sour cream. Top with the black olives and sliced scallions. Serve with chips or warmed pita bread for dipping.

NUTRITIONAL ANALYSIS

EACH WITH: Calories: 173.55, Protein: 8.90 g, Carbs: 18.41 g, Total Fat: 8.22 g, Sat Fat: 2.88 g, Cholesterol: 10.96 mg, Sodium: 466.05 mg, Sugars: 2.70 g, Fiber: 6.53 g,

CHAPTER 5

Vegetables and Side Dishes

Easy Broccoli and Cottage Cheese Casserole

TEXTURE: SOFT

2 cups (475 ml) water

3 cups (210 g) fresh broccoli florets

16 ounces (455 g) cottage cheese, 1% fat, no added salt

¾ cup (85 g) reduced-fat shredded Cheddar cheese

1 cup (160 g) diced yellow onion

3 egg whites, plus one whole egg, beaten

3 tablespoons (15 g) grated Parmesan cheese

—
Yield: Makes 6 (about ¾-cup) servings

Preheat the oven to 375°F (190°C, or gas mark 5). Coat a 9-inch (22.5-cm) pie pan or a 7- x 9-inch (17.5- x 22.5-cm) casserole dish with cooking spray.

In a 1½-quart (1.5-L) saucepan, bring the water to boil. Boil the broccoli for about 4 minutes, until al dente or still crunchy in the middle. Pour the broccoli into a colander and drain well.

In a medium size mixing bowl, combine the cottage cheese, Cheddar cheese, onion, egg, and Parmesan cheese. Pour the mixture into the pie pan or baking dish and bake for 35 to 45 minutes, until the center of the casserole is set. Allow the casserole to cool for about 10 minutes before serving.

NUTRITIONAL ANALYSIS

EACH WITH: Calories: 149.07, Protein: 18.13 g, Carbs: 7.89 g, Total Fat: 5.43 g, Sat Fat: 3.05 g, Cholesterol: 52.35 mg, Sodium: 229.95 mg, Sugars: 4.81 g, Fiber: 0.37 g

Brussels Hash

A delicious and new way to serve delicious Brussels sprouts.

TEXTURE: REGULAR

1 tablespoon (14 ml) olive oil

1½ cups (240 g) finely diced white onion

1 fresh clove garlic, minced

1 pound (455 g) Brussels sprouts, trimmed of stems and minced

1 tablespoon (10 g) finely chopped red bell pepper

½ cup (120 ml) low-sodium vegetable broth

½ teaspoon salt

⅛ teaspoon fresh cracked black pepper

—

Yield: Makes 6 (about ½-cup) servings

In a large skillet, heat the oil over medium heat. Add the onion and sauté, stirring frequently, for 5 minutes until it begins to soften. Add the garlic, Brussels sprouts, and bell pepper. Add the broth and simmer the vegetables, stirring occasionally, 5 to 8 minutes, until the broth has completely evaporated. Stir in the salt and black pepper. Sauté the hash another minute and serve.

NUTRITIONAL ANALYSIS

EACH WITH: Calories: 68.84, Protein: 3.17 g, Carbs: 6.41 g, Total Fat: 3.43 g, Sat Fat: 0.57 g, Cholesterol: 0.00 mg, Sodium: 106.79 mg, Sugars: 3.43 g, Fiber: 3.96 g

Creamy Polenta with Fresh Oregano and Feta Cheese

TEXTURE: SOFT

Polenta is as versatile as it is easy and delicious. It can be served as a side dish, and it also stands on its own as an entrée when paired with your favorite tomato sauce. Try some of the variations listed below.

1 cup (140 g) dry polenta meal (not corn meal)

1 cup (235 ml) nonfat milk

2½ cups (570 ml) water

⅛ teaspoon salt

2 tablespoons (8 g) chopped fresh oregano leaves

⅓ cup (50 g) feta cheese crumbles

—

Yield: Makes 8 (about ½-cup) servings

VARIATIONS

In place of water, use low-sodium chicken broth. In place of oregano and feta cheese, use ¼ cup (25 g) chopped green onion and ⅓ cup (40 g) reduced-fat, shredded Cheddar cheese, or ¼ cup (4 g) chopped fresh cilantro and 2 tablespoons (28 ml) lime juice, or 2 tablespoons (12 g) chopped green chilies and ⅓ cup (40 g) reduced-fat shredded Cheddar cheese. Or add 1 tablespoon (5 g) shredded Parmesan cheese.

Spray an 8- or 9-inch (20- or 22.5-cm) pie pan, a 7- x 7-inch (17.5- x 17.5-cm) baking dish, or sheet pan with cooking spray.

In a small bowl, place the polenta and pour the milk over the top. Stir the mixture to expose all the polenta to the liquid. (This process will eliminate lumps in the finished product.)

In a 1½-quart (1.5-L) saucepan, bring the water and salt to a soft boil and slowly add the soaked polenta, stirring constantly. Continue cooking, stirring, until the polenta begins to pull away from the sides of the pan. Remove the pan from the heat and stir in the oregano and cheese.

Immediately pour the polenta into the prepared pie pan or baking dish or spoon it free-form into a mound in the center of the sheet pan. Allow the polenta to cool until it sets enough to cut into squares or wedges (if serving from the free-form) and lifts away from the pan in one piece.

NUTRITIONAL ANALYSIS

EACH WITH: Calories: 125.51, Protein: 4.42 g, Carbs: 23.82 g, Total Fat: 1.46 g, Sat Fat: 0.99 g, Cholesterol: 6.18 mg, Sodium: 104.50 mg, Sugars: 1.77 g, Fiber: 1.12 g

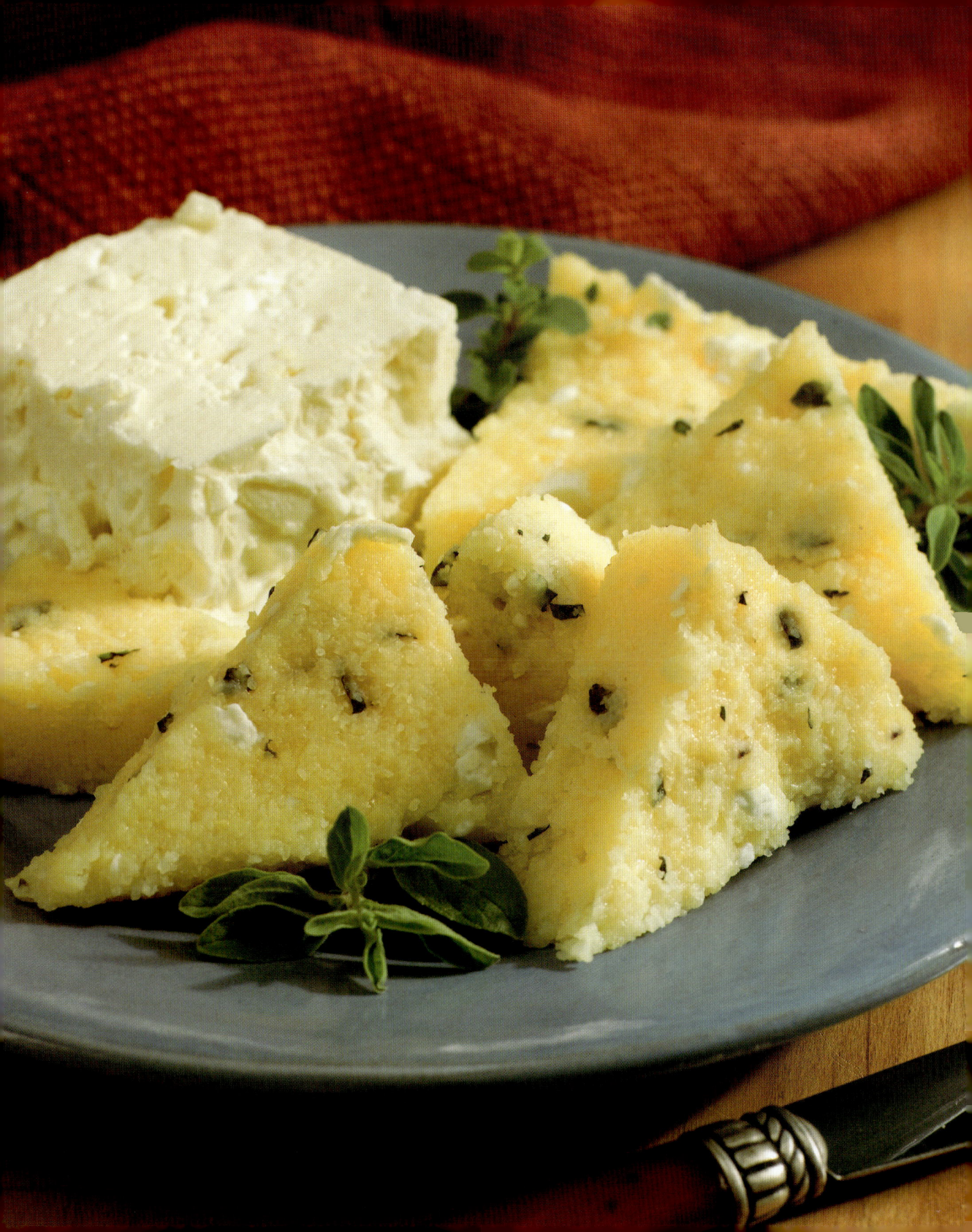

Parmesan Cheese and Green Pea Couscous

TEXTURE: MECHANICAL SOFT

Mmm ... this is so good! You have to try it!

1 can (14 ounces, or 425 ml) low-sodium chicken broth

¼ (60 ml) cup water

2 teaspoons extra-virgin olive oil

1 cup (175 g) whole-wheat couscous

1½ cups (195 g) frozen peas

2 tablespoons (8 g) fresh dill, chopped

1 teaspoon fresh lemon zest

1 teaspoon kosher salt

½ teaspoon black pepper

½ cup (50 g) fresh grated Parmesan cheese

—

Yield: Makes 8 (about ¼-cup) servings

Bring the chicken broth, water, and olive oil to a boil in a large saucepan. Stir in the couscous and remove from heat. Cover and allow the couscous to absorb the liquid for 5 minutes.

While couscous is "cooking," cook the peas according to the package directions. Add the cooked peas, dill, lemon zest, salt, and pepper to the couscous. Mix gently and fluff with a fork. Sprinkle with the Parmesan cheese and serve immediately.

NUTRITIONAL ANALYSIS

EACH WITH: Calories: 144.29, Protein: 7.13 g, Carbs: 22.20 g, Total Fat: 3.42 g, Sat Fat: 1.29 g, Cholesterol: 6.25 mg, Sodium: 448.74 mg, Sugars: 0.50 g, Fiber: 4.15 g

Heather's Ratatouille

TEXTURE: REGULAR

This hearty recipe comes from Heather, a gastric bypass surgery patient in the Boston area.

2 medium eggplants, peeled and cut into ½-inch (1.25-cm) cubes

2 medium zucchini, thinly sliced

½ teaspoon kosher salt

2 tablespoons (30 ml) extra-virgin olive oil

2 medium Vidalia onions, chopped

1 red bell pepper, seeded and cut into strips

1 yellow bell pepper, seeded and cut into strips

1 orange bell pepper, seeded and cut into strips

3 hot-house tomatoes, seeded and quartered

1 clove garlic, crushed

2 tablespoons (3 g) dried herbs de Provence

¼ teaspoon black pepper

—

Yield: Makes 12 (¾-cup) servings

Place the eggplant and zucchini in a colander and sprinkle with salt. Let drain for 30 to 60 minutes. Rinse with water then pat dry with a paper towel.

In a large skillet, heat the olive oil over medium heat. Add the onions and cook until translucent, about 6 minutes, stirring occasionally. Remove from the skillet and put in a large bowl.

In turn, cook the eggplant, zucchini, and peppers in the olive oil. When each vegetable is cooked, add it to the bowl. When all the vegetables are cooked, mix them together back in the skillet and add the tomatoes, garlic, herbs de Provence, and black pepper. Heat through and serve.

NUTRITIONAL ANALYSIS

EACH WITH: Calories: 50.07, Protein: 1.75 g, Carbs: 10.05 g, Total Fat: 1.02 g, Sat Fat: 0.16 g, Cholesterol: 0.00 mg, Sodium: 96.96 mg, Sugars: 5.14 g, Fiber: 3.89 g

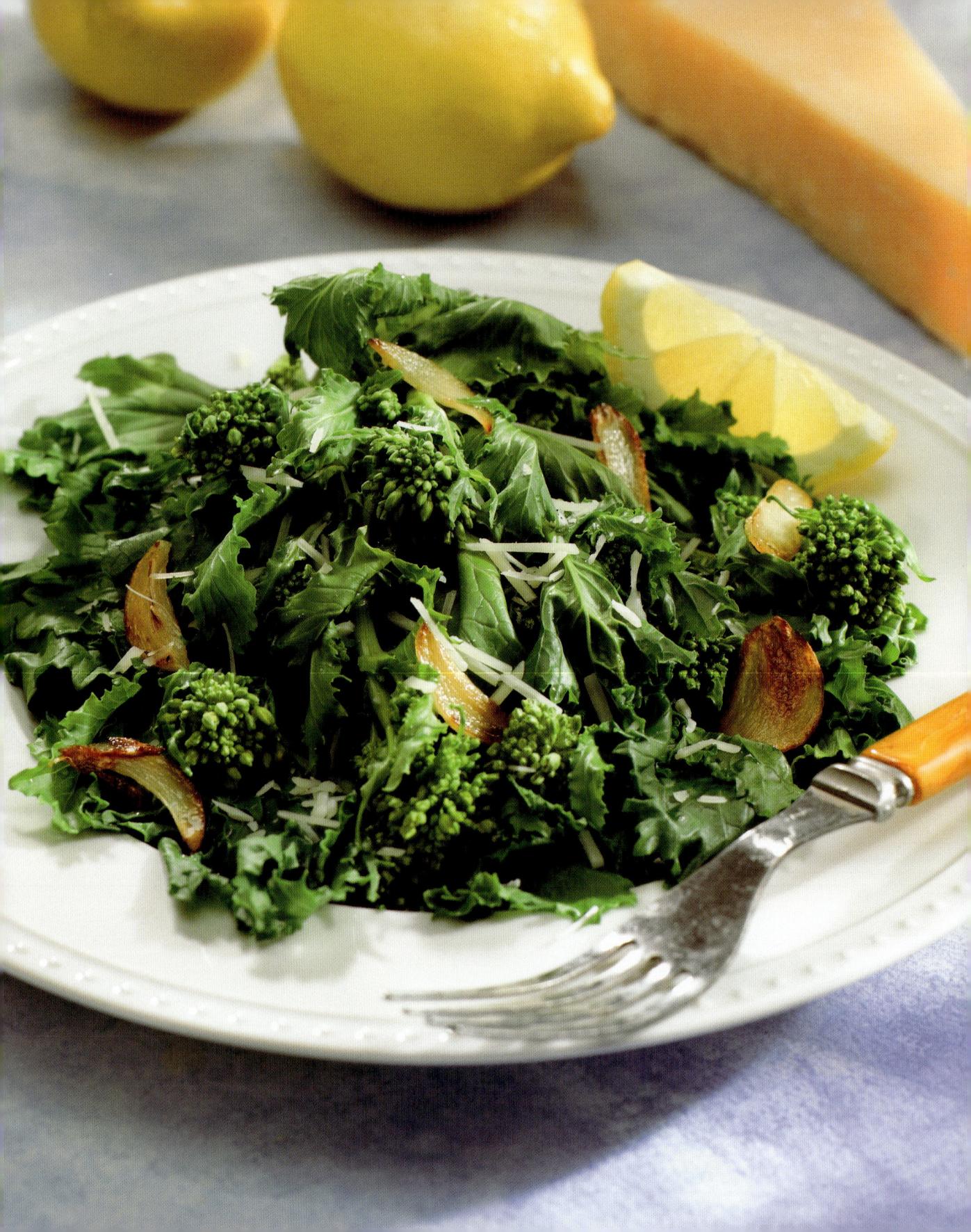

Broccoli Rabe

TEXTURE: REGULAR

Delicious, simple, and highly nutritious, this vegetable is a wonderful complement to fish or chicken.

4 cups (1 L) water

1 tablespoon (14 ml) extra-virgin olive oil

1 clove fresh garlic, cut into thin strips

1 pound (455 g) broccoli rabe, trimmed

2 teaspoons fresh lemon juice

⅛ teaspoon salt

⅛ teaspoon white pepper

1 teaspoon reduced-fat butter substitute

1 tablespoon (5 g) grated Parmesan cheese

—

Yield: Makes 4 (about ½-cup) servings

In a 1½-quart (1.5-L) saucepan, bring the water to a boil.

In a medium skillet, heat the oil over medium-high heat. Add the garlic and sauté until it just begins to brown. Immediately remove the garlic from the skillet and place it in a medium mixing bowl.

Add the broccoli rabe to the boiling water and cook for 2 to 3 minutes or until broccoli rabe is al dente, or still crunchy on the inside.

Place the lemon juice, salt, pepper, butter substitute, and cheese in the mixing bowl along with the garlic. Drain the broccoli rabe and add it to the bowl. Gently toss the broccoli rabe with the sauce. Serve immediately.

NUTRITIONAL ANALYSIS

EACH WITH: Calories: 71.08, Protein: 4.41 g, Carbs: 3.74 g, Total Fat: 5.12 g, Sat Fat: 1.02 g, Cholesterol: 0.75 mg, Sodium: 109.14 mg, Sugars: 0.45 g, Fiber: 3.10 g

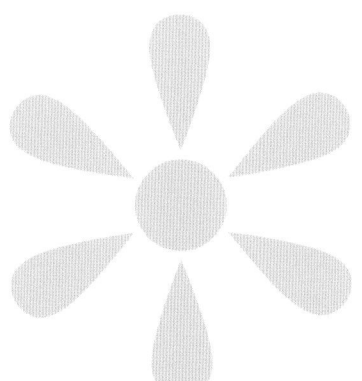

Chana Dal

TEXTURE: SOFT

This traditional dish from India is so delicious, you'll find yourself craving it after you've made it just once. Serve this in warm bowls with a dollop of plain low-fat yogurt and a sprinkle of fresh cilantro on top and Indian Papadum crackers on the side.

5 cups (1,175 ml) water

2 cups (400 g) chana dal (an Indian bean) or split yellow peas

1 medium yellow onion, finely diced

1 tablespoon (8 g) fresh grated gingerroot

1 tablespoon (10 g) fresh minced garlic (about 3 large cloves)

1 teaspoon ground coriander

1 teaspoon turmeric

1 teaspoon garam masala

1 tablespoon (16 g) tomato paste

2 tablespoons (28 ml) olive oil

2 teaspoons mustard seeds

1 teaspoon cumin seeds

1 small red chili pepper

½ teaspoon sea salt

¼ teaspoon white pepper

1 tablespoon (14 ml) fresh lemon juice

6 fresh cilantro sprigs, chopped

—
Yield: Makes 8 (about 1-cup) servings

In a 2½-quart (2.5-L) saucepan, bring the water, the chana dal or peas, onion, gingerroot, and garlic to a boil. Reduce the heat to medium-low and stir in the coriander, turmeric, garam masala, and tomato paste. Simmer uncovered for about 15 minutes, stirring occasionally.

When the chana dal is almost done (soft but not paste-like), heat the oil in a medium skillet along with the mustard seeds, cumin seeds, and chili pepper. Cook on medium-high for 1 to 2 minutes, until the seeds begin to crackle. Remove the chili pepper; add the seeds to the dal and stir in the salt, white pepper, and lemon juice. Garnish with cilantro sprigs.

NUTRITIONAL ANALYSIS

EACH WITH: Calories: 222.10, Protein: 12.79 g, Carbs: 33.72 g, Total Fat: 4.48 g, Sat Fat: 0.60 g, Cholesterol: 0.00 mg, Sodium: 150.67 mg, Sugars: 5.30 g, Fiber: 13.42 g

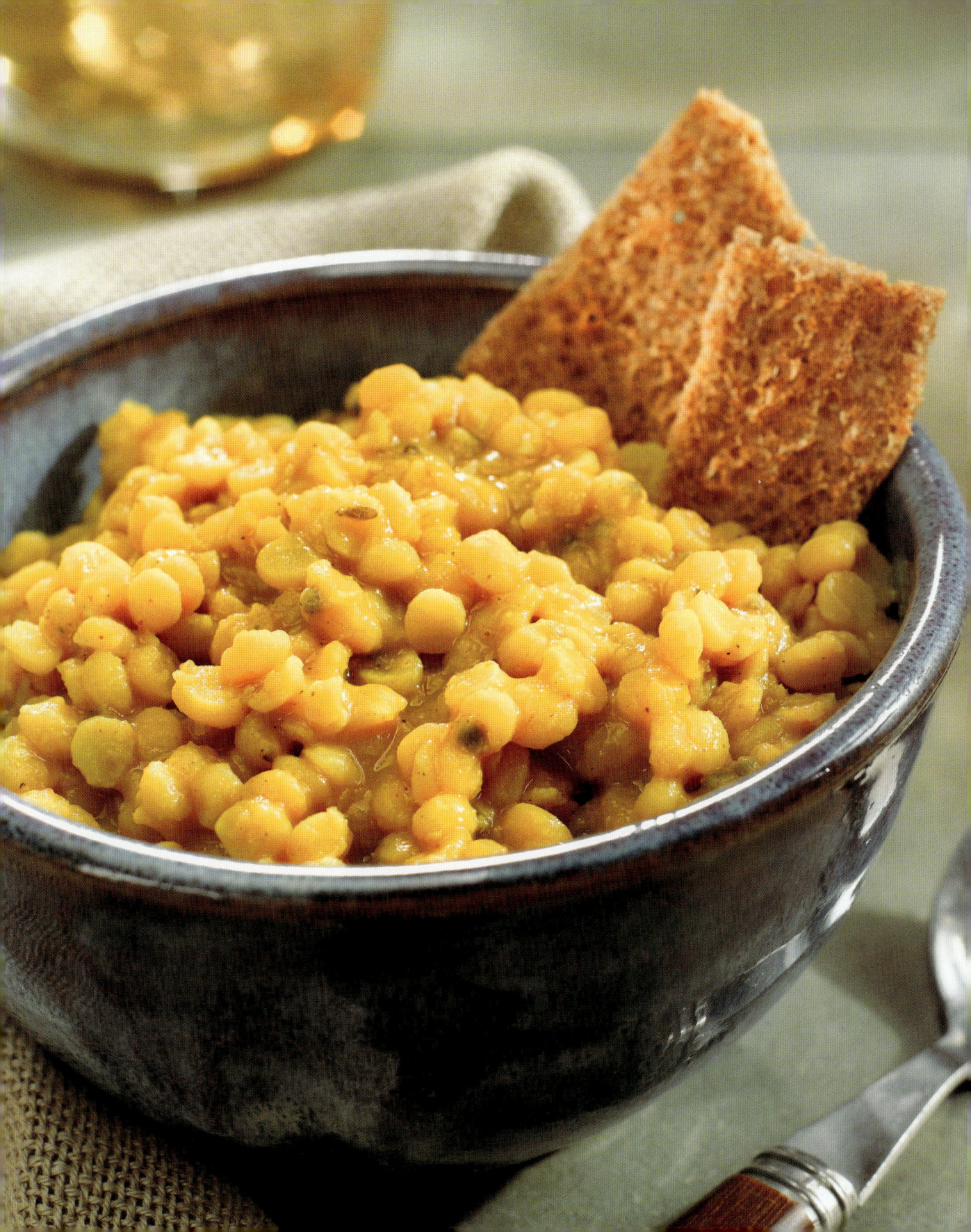

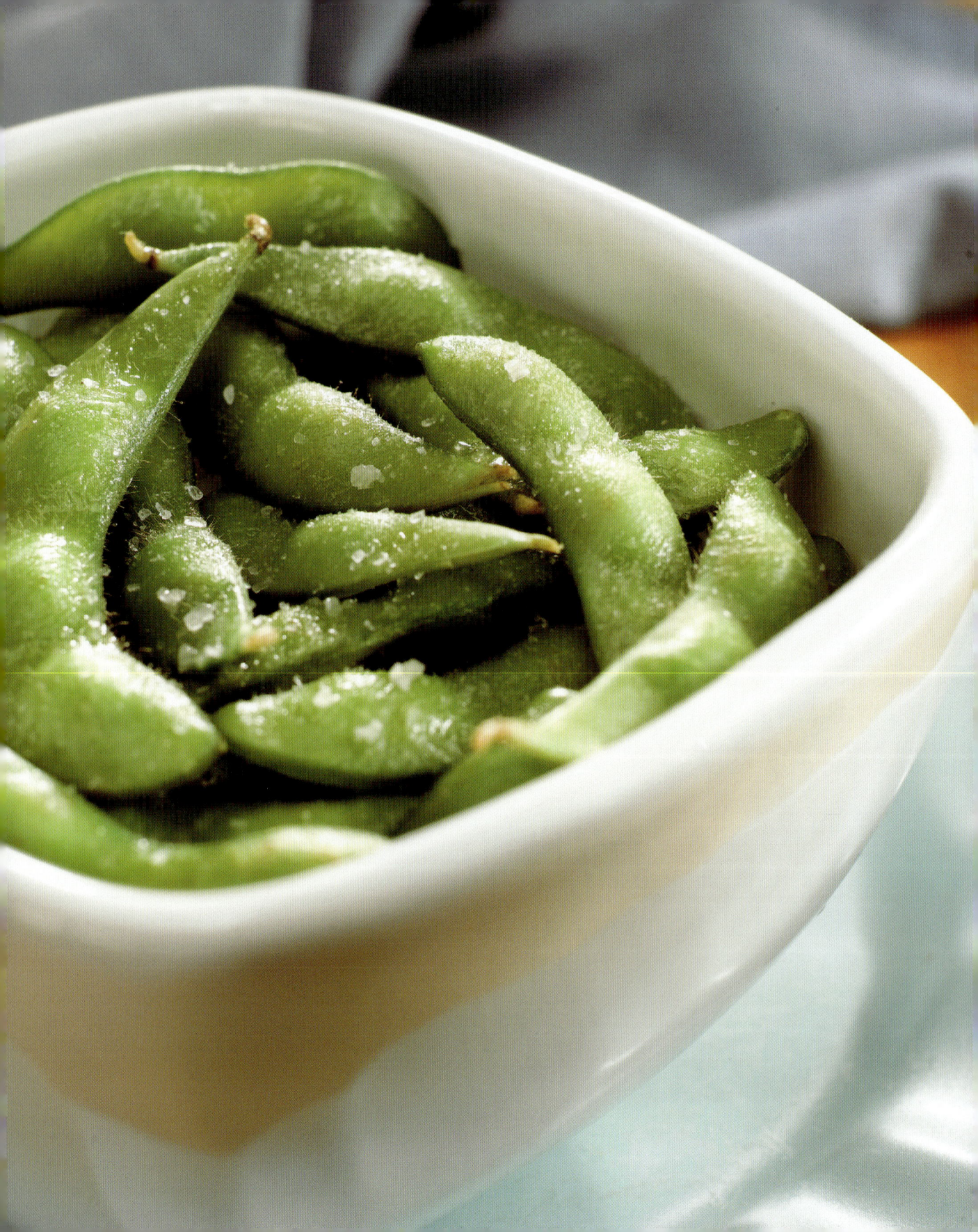

Edamame

TEXTURE: REGULAR

Edamame, whole soybeans in the shell, is a simple and nutritious way to get more soy protein in your diet. Pop the shells open and eat the beans inside. You can find them fresh or frozen at your grocer.

2½ quarts (2.5 L) water

1 tablespoon (18 g) salt

2 pounds (1 kg) fresh or frozen edamame

⅛ teaspoon coarse sea salt

—

Yield: Makes 14 (about 1-cup) servings

In a 3-quart (3-L) pot, bring the water and table salt to a boil over high heat. Add the edamame, reduce the heat, and simmer for 3 minutes if using fresh beans or 4 minutes if using frozen.

Drain the beans and transfer them to a serving bowl just large enough to hold the edamame. (If the serving container is too large, the beans will cool off too quickly.) Toss the beans with the coarse sea salt and serve immediately.

NUTRITIONAL ANALYSIS

EACH WITH: Calories: 91.48, Protein: 7.62 g, Carbs: 6.86 g, Total Fat: 3.81 g, Sat Fat: 0.38 g, Cholesterol: 0.00 mg, Sodium: 29.85 mg, Sugars: 2.29 g, Fiber: 3.05 g

Zesty Cajun Black-Eyed Peas

TEXTURE: REGULAR

2 cans (15½ ounces, or 439 g each) black-eyed peas, rinsed and drained

2 cups (454 g) canned crushed tomatoes

1 cup (235 ml) water

1 teaspoon low-sodium chicken bouillon granules, or 1 cube

1 large Vidalia onion, chopped

2 stalks celery, chopped

2 cloves garlic, minced

½ teaspoon dry mustard

¼ teaspoon ground ginger

¼ teaspoon cayenne pepper

1 bay leaf

⅛ cup (8 g) roughly chopped fresh parsley

—

Yield: Makes 8 (about 1-cup) servings

Combine the black-eyed peas, tomatoes, water, bouillon, onion, celery, garlic, mustard, ginger, cayenne pepper, and bay leaf in a large saucepan. Cover and simmer over medium-low heat for 2 hours, stirring occasionally. Add water as necessary to keep peas covered with liquid.

Remove the bay leaf and serve garnished with the parsley.

NUTRITIONAL ANALYSIS

EACH WITH: Calories: 131.68, Protein: 6.13 g, Carbs: 26.27 g, Total Fat: 0.17 g, Sat Fat: 0.04 g, Cholesterol: 0.03 mg, Sodium: 685.50 mg, Sugars: 4.95 g, Fiber: 5.67 g,

Herb and Cheese Mashed Cauliflower

Try this delicious and unique variation of cauliflower the whole family is sure to love.

2½ cups (570 ml) water

3 cups (450 g) cauliflower florets (about 1-inch, or 2.5-cm pieces)

⅔ cup (155 ml) nonfat milk

¼ cup (50 g) nonfat sour cream

½ teaspoon salt

⅛ teaspoon ground white pepper

2 tablespoons (15 g) finely chopped green onion

1 tablespoon (4 g) finely chopped fresh parsley

1 tablespoon (14 g) butter substitute

—

Yield: Makes 4 (about 1-cup) servings

In a 2½-quart (2.5-L) saucepan with a steamer basket, bring the water to a boil. Place the cauliflower in the steamer basket and steam for about 15 minutes, until the cauliflower is very tender throughout.

Place the cauliflower in a food processor fitted with a metal S blade and puree until smooth.

Add the milk and sour cream and carefully pulse the mixture until smooth. (Pulsate the mixture briefly to avoid the liquids splashing out of the processing bowl.) Add the salt, white pepper, onion, parsley, and butter substitute and continue pulsating until evenly incorporated. Serve warm as a side dish.

NUTRITIONAL ANALYSIS

EACH WITH: Calories: 88.13, Protein: 5.85 g, Carbs: 14.28 g, Total Fat: 1.76 g, Sat Fat: 0.35 g, Cholesterol: 3.32 mg, Sodium: 251.67 mg, Sugars: 7.13 g, Fiber: 4.41 g

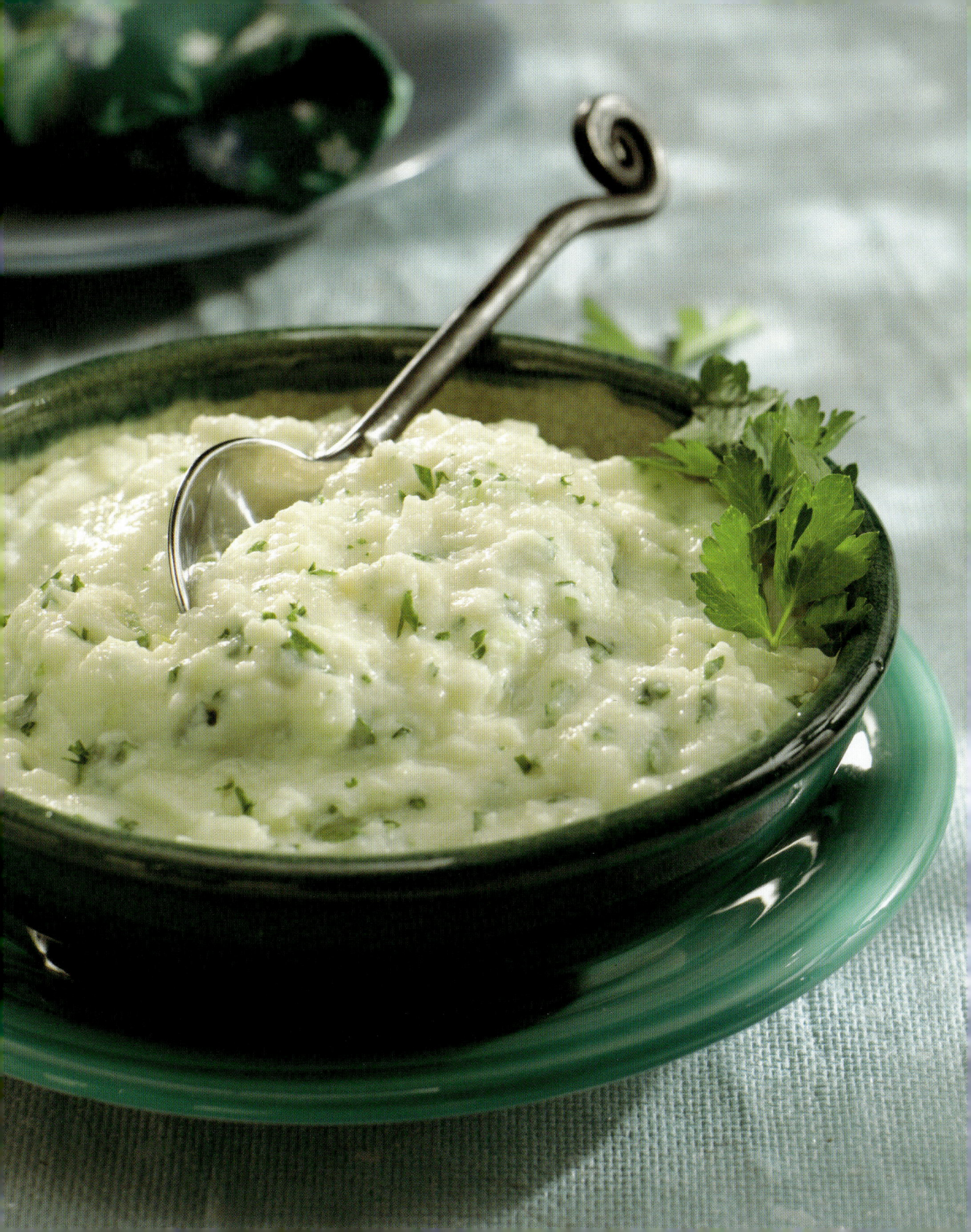

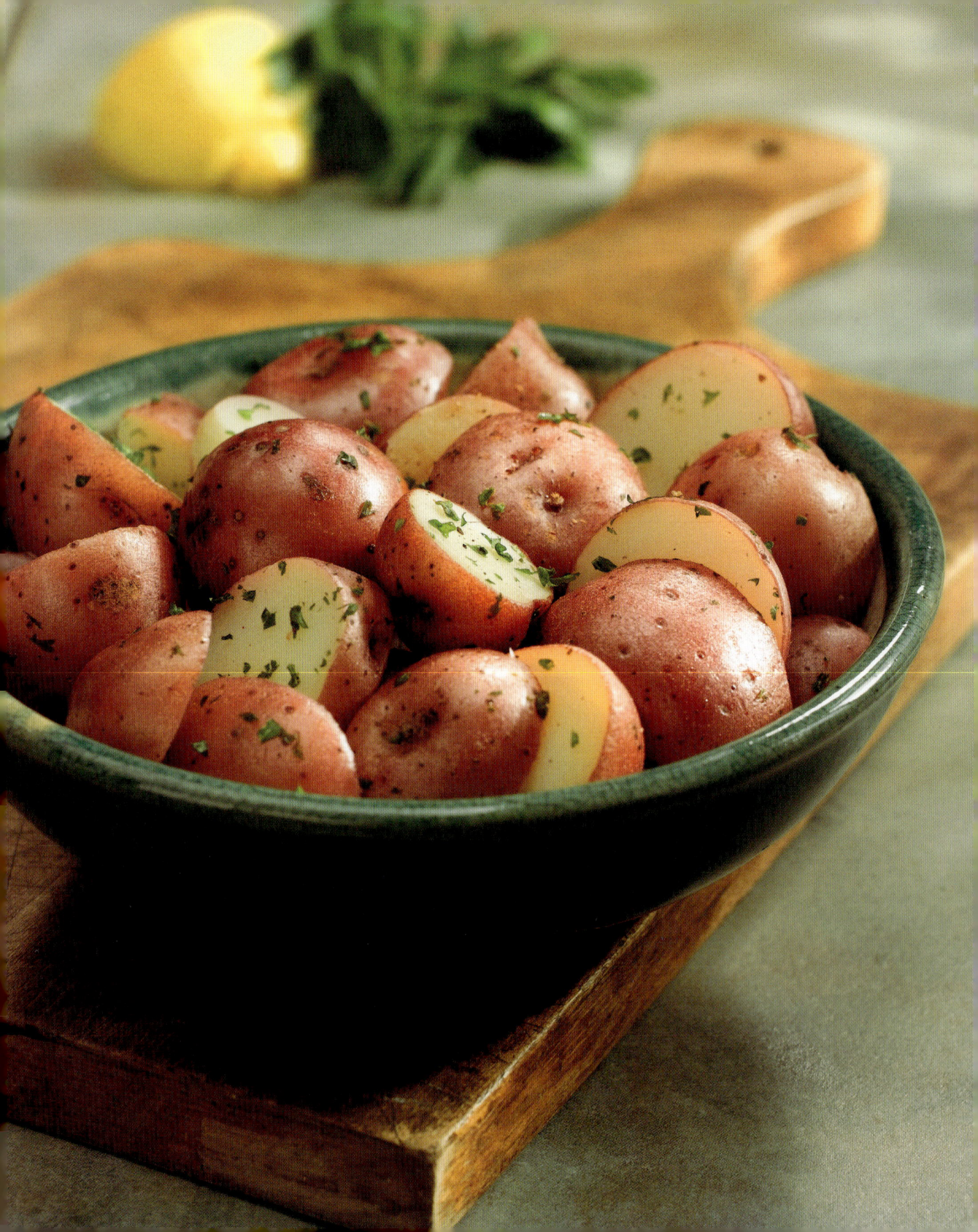

Boiled New Potatoes with Fresh Parsley

TEXTURE: SOFT

Pure, unadulterated deliciousness—this is a wonderful complement to roasted meat dishes.

1 pound (455 g) baby red potatoes, washed and halved

1 tablespoon (14 g) butter substitute

¼ teaspoon kosher salt

¼ teaspoon fresh cracked pepper

½ teaspoon fresh lemon juice

2 tablespoons (8 g) chopped fresh parsley

—
Yield: Makes 4 (about ½-cup) servings

In a 2-quart (2-L) saucepan, place the potatoes and enough cold water to cover 1 inch (2.5 cm) above the level of the potatoes. Bring the water to a boil and cook for about 12 minutes, until the potatoes can be gently speared with a fork when tested. Drain the potatoes in a colander and transfer them to a medium mixing bowl. While the potatoes are still hot, add the butter substitute, salt, pepper, lemon juice, and parsley. Gently toss the potatoes to evenly cover with all ingredients. Serve immediately.

NUTRITIONAL ANALYSIS

EACH WITH: Calories: 95.42, Protein: 2.23 g, Carbs: 18.28 g, Total Fat: 1.67 g, Sat Fat: 0.28 g, Cholesterol: 0.00 mg, Sodium: 147.87 mg, Sugars: 1.17 g, Fiber: 2.02 g

Sweet Potatoes au Gratin

TEXTURE: SOFT

1 tablespoon (14 g) light butter

1 medium onion, finely diced

1 small clove fresh garlic, minced

2½ cups (570 ml) low-sodium vegetable broth

½ cup (50 g) green onions, finely chopped

¼ cup (15 g) chopped fresh parsley

1 cup (235 ml) nonfat milk

¼ teaspoon salt

⅛ teaspoon ground black pepper

3 medium sweet potatoes, peeled and thinly sliced (about 2½ pounds, 1.25 kg)

½ cup (55 g) shredded reduced-fat Cheddar cheese

¼ cup (20 g) shredded Parmesan cheese

—

Yield: Makes 16 (about ¾-cup) servings

Preheat the oven to 375°F (190°C, or gas mark 5). Coat a 9- x 13-inch (22.5- x 32.5-cm) baking dish with cooking spray.

In a 2-quart (2-L) saucepan, melt the butter substitute over medium heat. Add the onion and garlic and sauté until the onion begins to soften, about 5 minutes. Add the broth, green onion, parsley, milk, salt, and pepper and bring to a simmer. Cook until the liquid is reduced to about 2¾ cups (650 ml). Add the sweet potatoes and return to a simmer. Continue cooking for an additional 5 minutes.

Pour the mixture into the prepared baking dish and bake for about 35 minutes, until the potatoes are tender, basting the potatoes occasionally with the liquid in the dish. Top the dish evenly with the Cheddar and then the Parmesan and continue to bake for about 20 minutes, until the cheese is bubbly and golden brown.

NUTRITIONAL ANALYSIS

EACH WITH: Calories: 104.14, Protein: 3.96 g, Carbs: 17.54 g, Total Fat: 2.03 g, Sat Fat: 1.03 g, Cholesterol: 4.37 mg, Sodium: 116.62 mg, Sugars: 4.09 g, Fiber: 2.15 g

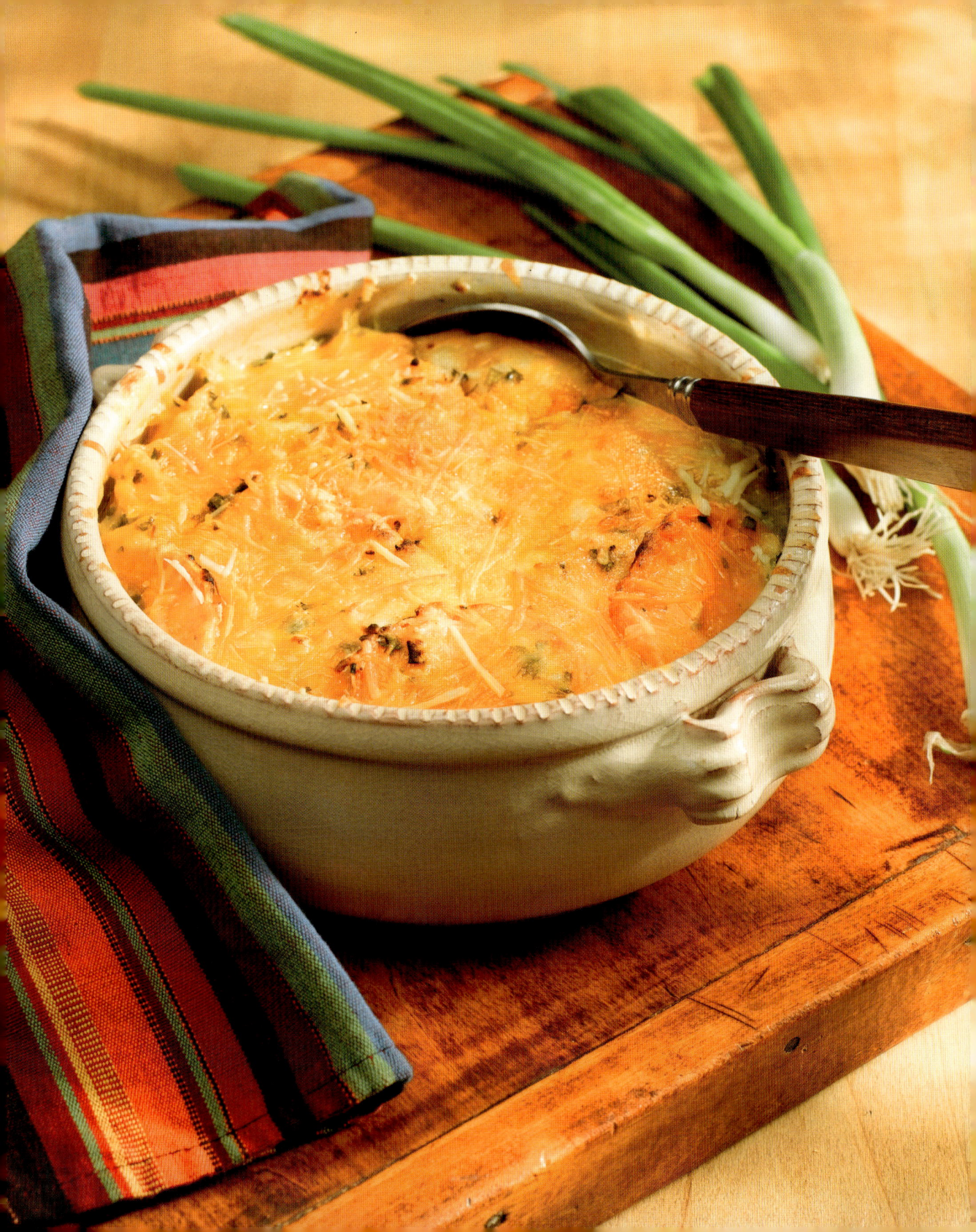

CHAPTER 6

Dinners

Pork Tenderloin Medallions with Spanish Smoked Paprika

TEXTURE: REGULAR

Hearts of Palm with Arugula and Endive Salad (page 67) makes the perfect accompaniment to this delicious and savory dish.

1 pound (455 g) pork tenderloin roast

1 tablespoon (14 ml) olive oil

2 tablespoons (28 ml) Worcestershire sauce

1 teaspoon Spanish smoked paprika

⅛ teaspoon ground white pepper

2 teaspoons light butter

—

Yield: Makes 4 (about 3-ounce) servings

Trim off any excess fat from the pork tenderloin and cut it into 1-inch (2.5-cm) medallions.

In a medium mixing bowl, combine the oil, Worcestershire sauce, paprika, and white pepper.

Place the pork in the bowl with the marinade and turn it a few times to coat the medallions evenly.

In a nonstick skillet, heat the butter over medium-high heat. Lay the pork medallions in the pan and cook 4 to 6 minutes, until browned on the first side. Turn and cook an additional 4 to 6 minutes, until the second side is browned. Remove the medallions from the pan and let rest for 5 minutes before serving.

NUTRITIONAL ANALYSIS

EACH WITH: Calories: 201.85, Protein: 25.01 g, Carbs: 2.37 g, Total Fat: 10.87 g, Sat Fat: 2.51 g, Cholesterol: 67.15 mg, Sodium: 65.22 mg, Sugars: 1.43 g, Fiber: 0.02 g

Cheddar Chipotle Beer Chicken

TEXTURE: REGULAR

2 tablespoons (28 ml) extra-virgin olive oil

6 (4-ounce, or 115 g) boneless, skinless chicken breasts

1 tablespoon (10 g) chopped garlic

1 bottle (12 ounces, or 355 ml) beer of your choosing

½ cup (120 ml) skim milk

1 tablespoon chipotle powder

1 slice (1 ounce, or 15 g) low-fat Cheddar cheese

—
Yield: Makes 6 (about 6½-ounce) servings

Heat the olive oil in a medium skillet over medium heat. Sear the chicken until golden brown, about 3 minutes on both sides.

Add the garlic to the pan and sauté for about 1 to 2 minutes. Add the beer, milk, and chipotle powder to the pan. Bring to a simmer, then reduce until the liquid has reached a sauce-like consistency. Remove the pan from the heat and stir in the Cheddar cheese until it is completely incorporated in the sauce.

NUTRITIONAL ANALYSIS

EACH WITH: Calories: 283.05, Protein: 37.25 g, Carbs: 3.91 g, Total Fat: 9.98 g, Sat Fat: 2.39 g, Cholesterol: 100.13 mg, Sodium: 132.32 mg, Sugars: 1.01 g, Fiber: 0.00 g

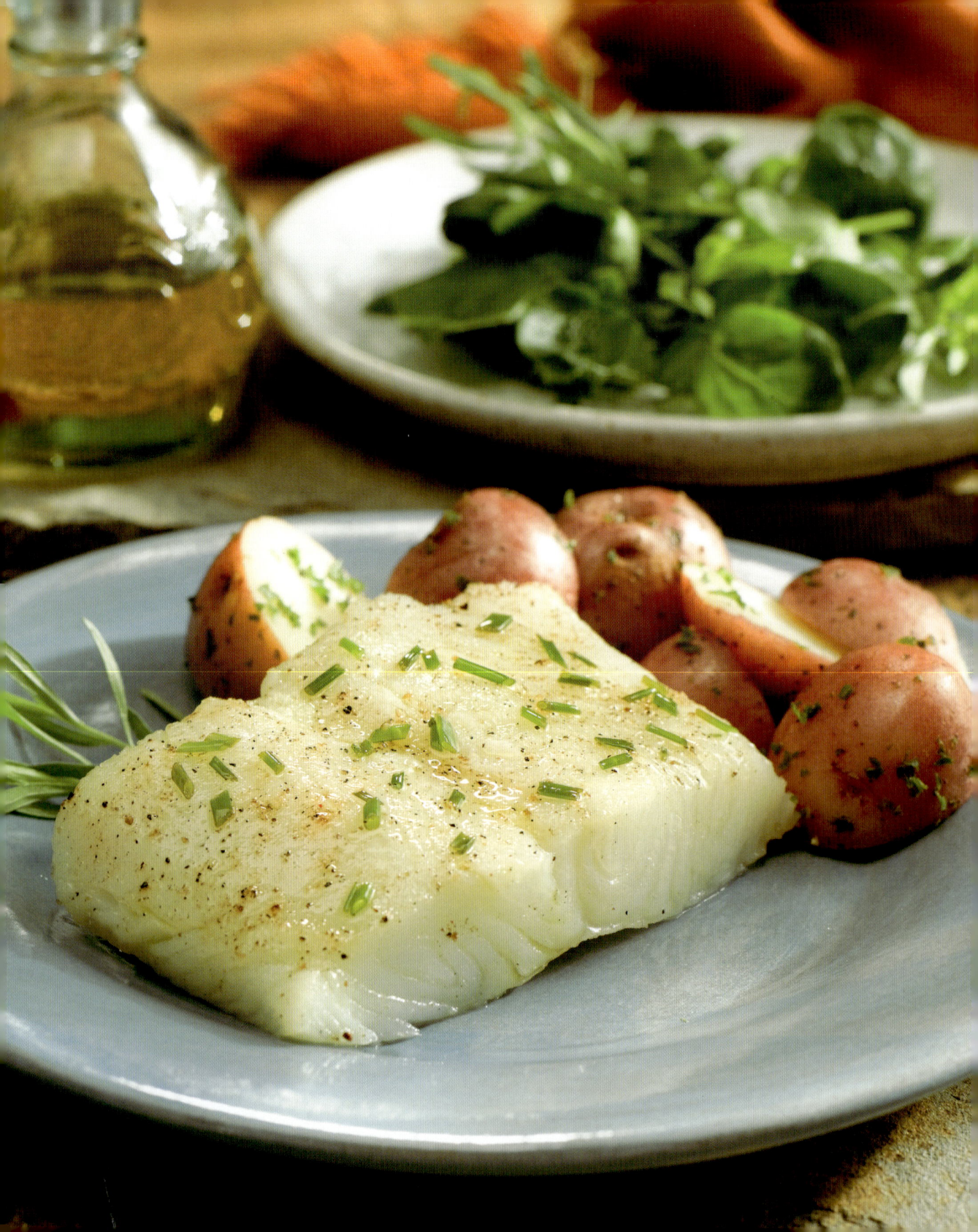

Baked Sea Bass

TEXTURE: SOFT

This is as easy as it is delicious. Impress your friends with this recipe at your next dinner party.

1¼ pounds (570 g) sea bass

½ teaspoon sea salt or kosher salt

¼ teaspoon white pepper

¼ teaspoon black pepper

2 tablespoons (28 ml) extra-virgin olive oil

1 tablespoon (3 g) thinly sliced chives

2 tablespoons (28 ml) sherry wine for cooking or chicken broth

2 teaspoons fresh lemon juice

—

Yield: Makes 4 (about 6-ounce) servings

Cut the fillets into 4 equal servings and place them in a medium baking dish, skin sides down.

In a small bowl, combine the salt and white pepper and lightly coat both sides of the fillets. Sprinkle the top with the black pepper. Cover and let stand in refrigerator for 10 to 15 minutes.

In a small bowl, combine the oil, chives, sherry or broth, and lemon juice and briefly whisk with a fork or wire whisk. Spread the mixture evenly over the fillets and let stand for an additional 10 minutes.

Preheat the oven to 400°F (200°C, or gas mark 6) and bake the fillets about 7 minutes for every inch of thickness, until the center of the fillets are no longer translucent and the outsides of the fillets begin to flake when tested with a fork. Let the fillets stand and cool for about 3 minutes. With a metal spatula, remove the fillets by separating the flesh from the skin and place them in the center of a serving plate.

LYNETTE'S NOTE

Colorful garnishes for this plate include fresh, edible flowers, such as nasturtiums, lemon wedges, or fresh herb sprigs.

NUTRITIONAL ANALYSIS

EACH WITH: Calories: 207.43, Protein: 26.33 g, Carbs: 0.40 g, Total Fat: 9.87 g, Sat Fat: 1.73 g, Cholesterol: 58.12 mg, Sodium: 332.99 mg, Sugars: 0.13 g, Fiber: 0.14 g

Pot Roast à la Sara

TEXTURE: REGULAR

This meat, a specialty of my mom's, is so tender it melts in your mouth. You'll love it.

2 pounds (1 kg) beef bottom round roast

½ cup (120 ml) red wine or beef broth

½ cup (120 ml) water

4 large cloves garlic

1 bay leaf

1 teaspoon salt

1–2 jalapeño peppers (optional)

1½ tablespoons (21 ml) canola oil

½ pound (225 g) peeled and cubed Yukon Gold or baby red potatoes (cut into 1-inch, or 2.5-cm cubes)

½ pound (225 g) baby carrots, cleaned and trimmed

—

Yield: Makes 10 (about 3-ounce meat) servings

Place the beef, wine or broth, water, garlic, bay leaf, salt, and peppers (if using) in a baking dish. Marinate the beef for at least 15 minutes in the refrigerator.

In a 3- or 4-quart (3- or 4-L) heavy-bottomed pot, place the oil over medium-high heat. When the oil is hot, place the beef in the pot, reserving all of the marinade in a separate container. Brown the beef on all sides by allowing it to cook for about 4 to 5 minutes on each side, then rotating it with kitchen tongs or a serving fork. (The object here is to completely brown the entire surface of the roast in order to seal in the juices.) When the roast is nicely browned, add the remaining marinade and reduce the heat to low. Cover with a tight-fitting lid and cook for 1½ hours, until the beef is fork tender. Add the potatoes and carrots. Cook for an additional 1 to 1½ hours, until the potatoes and carrots are tender. Remove the bay leaf before serving.

NUTRITIONAL ANALYSIS

EACH WITH: Calories: 229.28, Protein: 19.56 g, Carbs: 6.87 g, Total Fat: 12.60 g, Sat Fat: 4.29 g, Cholesterol: 52.62 mg, Sodium: 183.65 mg, Sugars: 1.34 g, Fiber: 1.21 g

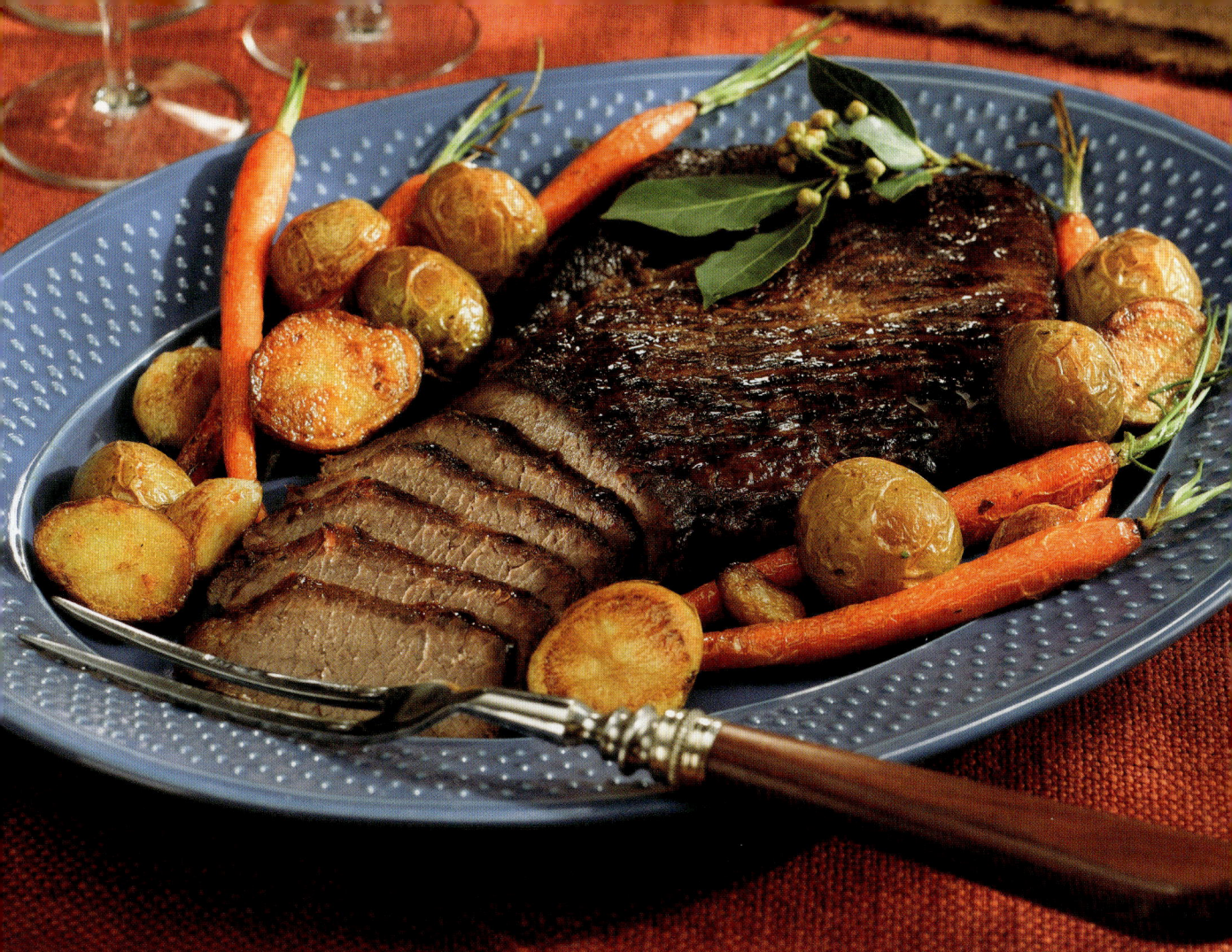

MARGARET'S NOTE

Although this dish is a bit higher in fat than fish or lean chicken, many weight-loss surgery patients may be able to tolerate a 3-ounce serving of this pot roast about 2 or 3 months postop, if not sooner. Eating mindfully (i.e. taking small, pencil-eraser-size bites and chewing at least 15 times prior to swallowing) should allow for better tolerance overall. If you find that meat, even a tender one like this pot roast, is a bit heavier for you, perhaps try only 2 ounces. As always, it's important to stop eating if you feel chest pressure or pain, which is typically your body's signal that you've had enough to eat at a particular sitting.

I hope you enjoy my mom's succulent pot roast dish! Thanks again, Mom!

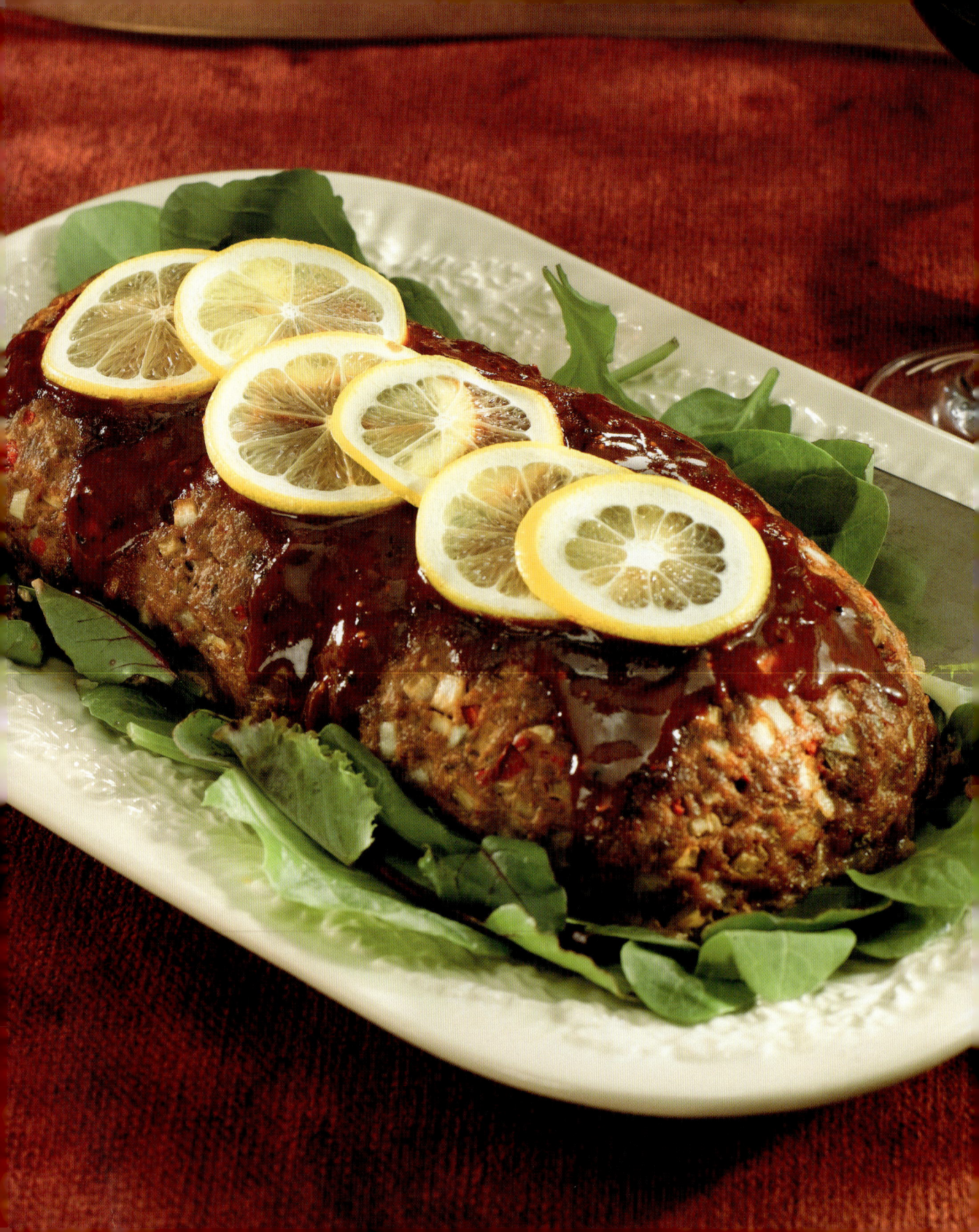

Lemon-Barbecue Meatloaf

TEXTURE: SOFT

This is a great dish for the family, or it can be easy divided and frozen for later.

2 pounds (1 kg) 95% lean ground beef

2 cups (320 g) diced yellow onion
(about 1½ onions)

2 tablespoons (28 ml) fresh lemon juice

7 tablespoons (105 ml) low-carb barbecue sauce,
divided

2 tablespoons (30 g) low-sodium tomato paste

2 tablespoons (8 g) chopped fresh parsley

¼ cup (35 g) finely chopped green
or red bell pepper

1 large egg

¼ cup (25 g) bread crumbs

6 ⅛ -inch (3 mm) thick lemon slices

—

**Yield: Makes 12 (about 3-ounce)
servings**

Preheat the oven to 375°F (190°C, or gas mark 5). Spray a 8½- x 13½-inch (22.5- x 32.5-cm) baking dish with cooking spray.

In a large mixing bowl, place the beef, onion, lemon juice, 4 tablespoons (60 ml) of the barbecue sauce, tomato paste, parsley, pepper, egg, and bread crumbs. Mix until well incorporated.

Form the mixture into a loaf and pat it down to condense the consistency. The loaf should touch the width, or short edges of the pan, but leave a few inches of room on both sides of the length.

Bake uncovered for 30 minutes. Remove the loaf from the oven and coat the top with the additional 3 tablespoons (45 ml) barbecue sauce. Place the lemon slices on top of the loaf and return it to the oven. Continue baking for an additional 20 minutes.

NUTRITIONAL ANALYSIS

EACH WITH: Calories: 170.19, Protein: 22.31 g, Carbs: 6.04 g, Total Fat: 5.79 g, Sat Fat: 2.43 g, Cholesterol: 75.21 mg, Sodium: 160.16 mg, Sugars: 1.91 g, Fiber: 0.88 g

Sausage with Lentils

TEXTURE: REGULAR

2 tablespoons (30 ml) extra-virgin olive oil

12 ounces (340 g) chicken sausage, thinly sliced

2 medium onions, chopped

2 red bell peppers, cored, seeded, and chopped

1 orange bell pepper, cored, seeded and chopped

1½ cups (290 g) small green lentils, rinsed

1 teaspoon dried thyme

2 cups (480 ml) low-fat, low-sodium chicken stock

½ teaspoon kosher salt

¼ teaspoon black pepper

4 tablespoons (16 g) fresh parsley, chopped

—

Yield: Makes 8 (about 1-cup) servings

Heat the olive oil in a large, nonstick skillet over medium-high heat. Add the sausage and cook, stirring frequently, about 10 minutes, or until the sausage is brown.

Pour off the oil from the skillet. Add the onions and bell peppers and cook for about 5 minutes, or until softened. Add the lentils and thyme, and stir until coated with oil.

Stir in the stock, and bring to a boil. Reduce the heat, cover, and let simmer for about 30 minutes, or until the lentils are tender and the liquid has been absorbed; season with salt and pepper.

Return the sausage to the skillet and heat through. Stir in the parsley before serving.

NUTRITIONAL ANALYSIS

EACH WITH: Calories: 232.47, Protein: 16.42 g, Carbs: 25.82 g, Total Fat: 7.70 g, Sat Fat: 1.33 g, Cholesterol: 31.89 mg, Sodium: 505.73 mg, Sugars: 4.52 g, Fiber: 6.81 g

Greek Yogurt-Cucumber Sauce

TEXTURE: PUREED

1 cup (135 g) grated cucumber (Squeeze out excess moisture using paper towels.)

½ cup (100 g) nonfat sour cream

1 container (7 ounces, or 200 g) 2% Greek yogurt

1 clove fresh garlic, minced

1 teaspoon lemon juice

¼ teaspoon salt

⅛ teaspoon ground white pepper

1 tablespoon (4 g) chopped fresh parsley

—

Yield: Makes 10 (about 1-ounce) servings

In a medium mixing bowl, stir together the cucumber, sour cream, yogurt, garlic, lemon juice, salt, pepper, and parsley with a wire whip. Serve chilled.

NUTRITIONAL ANALYSIS

EACH WITH: Calories: 29.40, Protein: 2.61 g, Carbs: 3.68 g, Total Fat: 0.43 g, Sat Fat: 0.30 g, Cholesterol: 3.00 mg, Sodium: 45.79 mg, Sugars: 1.80 g, Fiber: 0.12 g

"Braised" Lamb with Zucchini and Tomatoes

TEXTURE: REGULAR

12 ounces (340 g) lamb chops

½ teaspoon kosher salt

¼ teaspoon black pepper

2 tablespoons (30 ml) extra-virgin olive oil

1 medium onion, chopped

1 garlic clove, minced

1 can (14½ ounces, or 411 g) diced tomatoes, no salt added

¼ teaspoon sugar

2 medium zucchinis, sliced

1 teaspoon dried thyme

—

Yield: Makes 6 (about 6-ounce) servings

Season the lamb chops with salt and pepper. Heat the olive oil in a Dutch oven or large heavy-duty pot over medium-high heat. Add the onion and garlic and sauté for about 5 minutes, or until softened. Add the lamb chops and sear until brown, about 3 minutes on each side.

Stir in the tomatoes with juice, sugar, zucchini, and thyme. Bring to a boil and then turn the heat to medium-low and simmer, stirring occasionally, for 30 to 45 minutes, or until the zucchini and lamb chops are tender. Serve by topping the lamb chops with the vegetables and sauce.

NUTRITIONAL ANALYSIS

EACH WITH: Calories: 181.47, Protein: 15.97 g, Carbs: 5.62 g, Total Fat: 10.14 g, Sat Fat: 2.95 g, Cholesterol: 49.33 mg, Sodium: 214.29 mg, Sugars: 3.79 g, Fiber: 1.08 g

Slow-Cooked Sausage and Lentil Stew

Tasty and satisfying, this can be started in the morning and ready at dinnertime.

1½ cups (290 g) lentils, soaked in water for 30 minutes

½ cup (50 g) chopped celery

2 cups (40 g) chopped fresh spinach, washed and drained

3 cloves fresh garlic, coarsely chopped

1 cup (160 g) chopped yellow onion

4 cups (1 L) water

2 tablespoons (30 g) low-sodium tomato paste

½ teaspoon cayenne pepper (optional)

1 bay leaf

Juice of ½ lemon (about 2 tablespoons, or 28 ml)

½ pound (225 g) light, low-sodium precooked smoked turkey sausage or kielbasa, cut into ¼-inch (6-mm) pieces, skin removed (see note)

—

Yield: Makes 6 (about 1-cup) servings

In a 3-quart (3-L) slow cooker, place all ingredients and cook on the high setting for 5 hours or on the low setting for 7 hours. Remove the bay leaf before serving.

NUTRITIONAL ANALYSIS

EACH WITH: Calories: 261.32, Protein: 20.45 g, Carbs: 33.07 g, Total Fat: 6.01 g, Sat Fat: 0.09 g, Cholesterol: 23.33 mg, Sodium: 371.91 mg, Sugars: 4.87 g, Fiber: 15.98 g

NOTE

Removing the skin is essential for easier digestion. Score the sausage lengthwise and peel the skin away from the sausage. The skin will come right off.

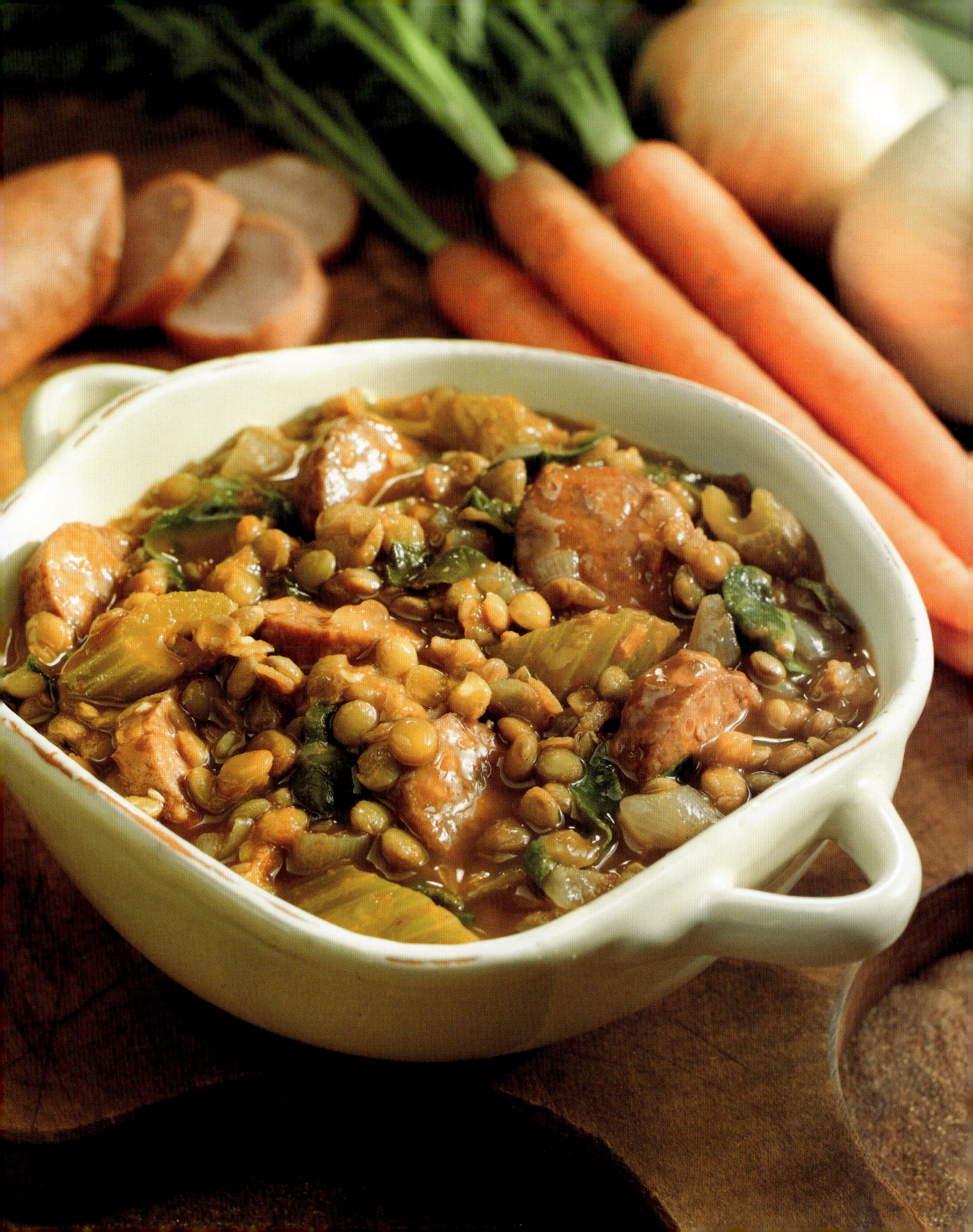

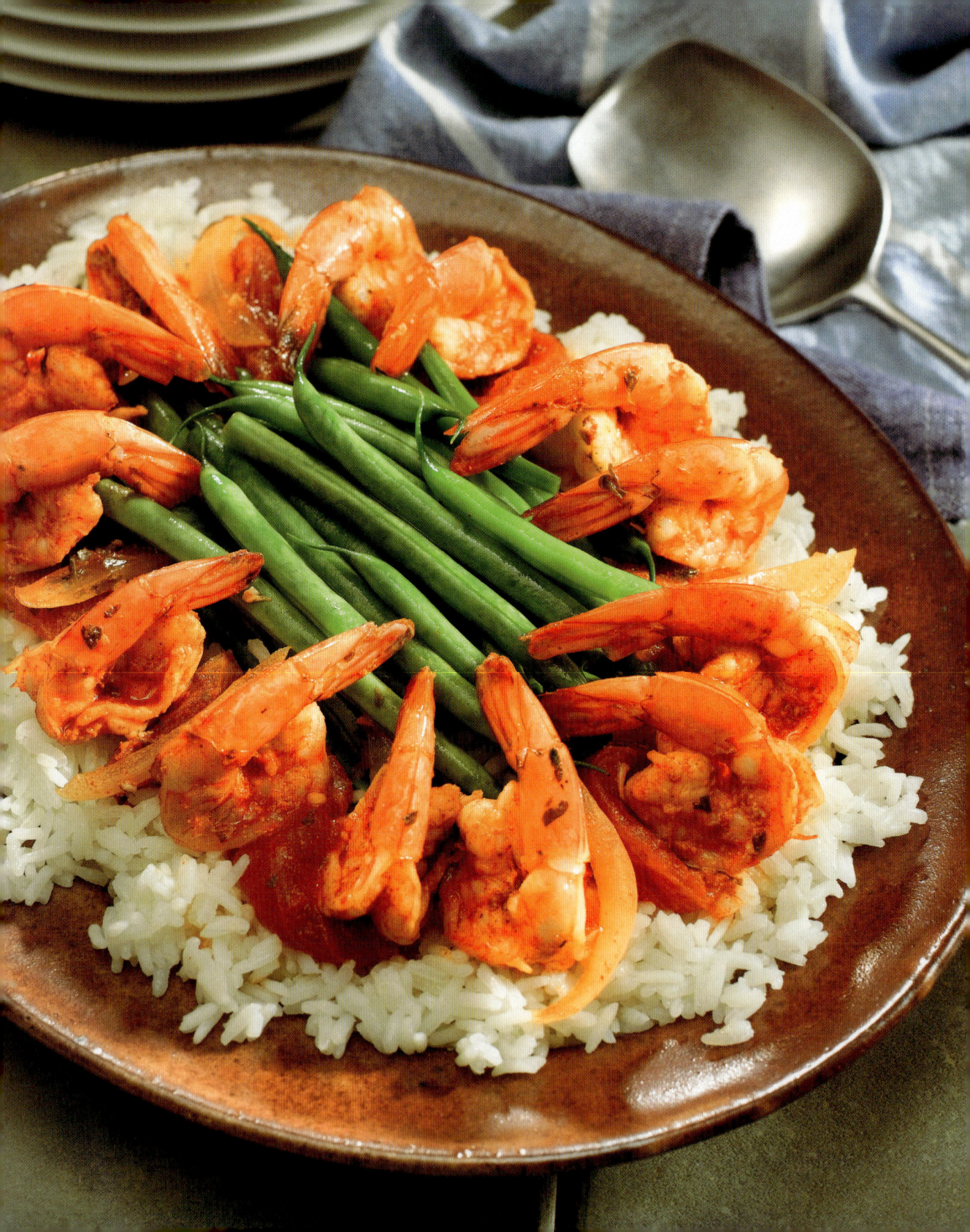

Spanish Shrimp with Jasmine Rice and Green Beans

TEXTURE: REGULAR

¾ cup (135 g) dry jasmine rice

1½ cups (355 ml) cold water

1 pound (455 g) fresh green beans

2 cups (475 ml) water

1 pound (455 g) medium to large fresh shrimp, peeled and deveined

½ teaspoon salt

¼ teaspoon black pepper

1 tablespoon (14 ml) extra-virgin olive oil

1 cup (160 g) julienned sweet onion (cut into ¼-inch (6-mm) strips

2 cloves fresh garlic, minced

1½ cups (290 g) quartered plum tomatoes, skins removed

½ cup (120 ml) sherry or chicken broth or vegetable broth

2 teaspoons dried oregano

1 teaspoon smoked Spanish paprika

⅛ teaspoon cayenne pepper (optional)

¼ cup (15 g) chopped fresh parsley

5 lemon wedges

—

Yield: Makes 5 (about 1-cup) servings

Rinse and drain the rice in cold water, then place it in a 1-quart (1-L) saucepan with the 1½ cups (355 ml) cold water. Bring the rice to a boil and then reduce the heat to a simmer. Continue to cook, loosely covered, for 20 minutes, until the water is absorbed by the rice.

Wash and drain the green beans. Snap off the stems and any remaining strings. In a 2½-quart (2.5-L) saucepan with a steamer basket, place the beans along with the 2 cups (475 ml) water. Cover and bring the water to a boil. Continue to steam the green beans for about 5 minutes, until the desired doneness is reached.

Butterfly the prawns by using a paring knife to score the backside of each one at a depth of about ¼ inch (6 mm). Place prawns on a plate or sheet pan in a single layer. Sprinkle the salt and pepper on the prawns and set aside.

In an 8-inch (20-cm) skillet, heat the oil over medium-high heat. When the oil is hot, add the onion and garlic and sauté for about 3 minutes, until the onion begins to soften. Add the tomatoes, sherry or broth, oregano, paprika, and cayenne pepper (if using). Reduce the heat to medium-low and continue cooking for 2 minutes. Add the prawns and cook about 5 minutes, until an orange color can be seen throughout each prawn. Remove from the heat.

Divide the rice among five dinner plates. Arrange the prawns around the rice so that the tails are facing upward. Sprinkle each plate with parsley. Arrange the steamed green beans asymmetrically around the prawns. Garnish each plate with a lemon wedge.

NUTRITIONAL ANALYSIS

EACH WITH: Calories: 296.73, Protein: 22.26 g, Carbs: 34.67 g, Total Fat: 4.76 g, Sat Fat: 0.74 g, Cholesterol: 137.89 mg, Sodium: 654.61 mg, Sugars: 5.89 g, Fiber: 3.67 g

Eggplant Parmesan

TEXTURE: SOFT

1 large eggplant (about 1¼ pounds, or 570 g)

½ teaspoon salt

1 tablespoon (14 ml) olive oil

½ cup (80 g) diced yellow onion

2 cans (11 ounces, or 310 g each) tomato sauce, no salt added

1 teaspoon dried basil

1 teaspoon dried oregano

¼ cup (15 g) chopped fresh parsley

1 teaspoon dried thyme

1 cup (110 g) part skim-milk mozzarella cheese

1 tablespoon (5 g) grated Parmesan cheese

—

Yield: Makes 6 (about 1-cup) servings

Preheat the oven to 375°F (190°C, or gas mark 5). Spray a 9- x 13-inch (22.5- x 32.5-cm) baking dish with cooking spray.

Remove the skin and stem from the eggplant with a vegetable peeler or a small kitchen knife.

Cut the eggplant into ¼-inch (6-mm) circles and arrange them overlapping in the prepared baking dish. Evenly sprinkle the eggplant slices with the salt. Drizzle the oil on top of the eggplant. Distribute the onions evenly on top of the eggplant. Pour the tomato sauce evenly on top of the eggplant, allowing it to disperse throughout the slices. Evenly sprinkle the basil, oregano, parsley, and thyme on top of the sauce. Spread the mozzarella and Parmesan over the top. Bake for 30 to 40 minutes, until the cheese is bubbly and golden brown.

NUTRITIONAL ANALYSIS

EACH WITH: Calories: 138.58, Protein: 6.85 g, Carbs: 14.72 g, Total Fat: 6.01 g, Sat Fat: 2.55 g, Cholesterol: 10.73 mg, Sodium: 233.87 mg, Sugars: 7.16 g, Fiber: 5.03 g

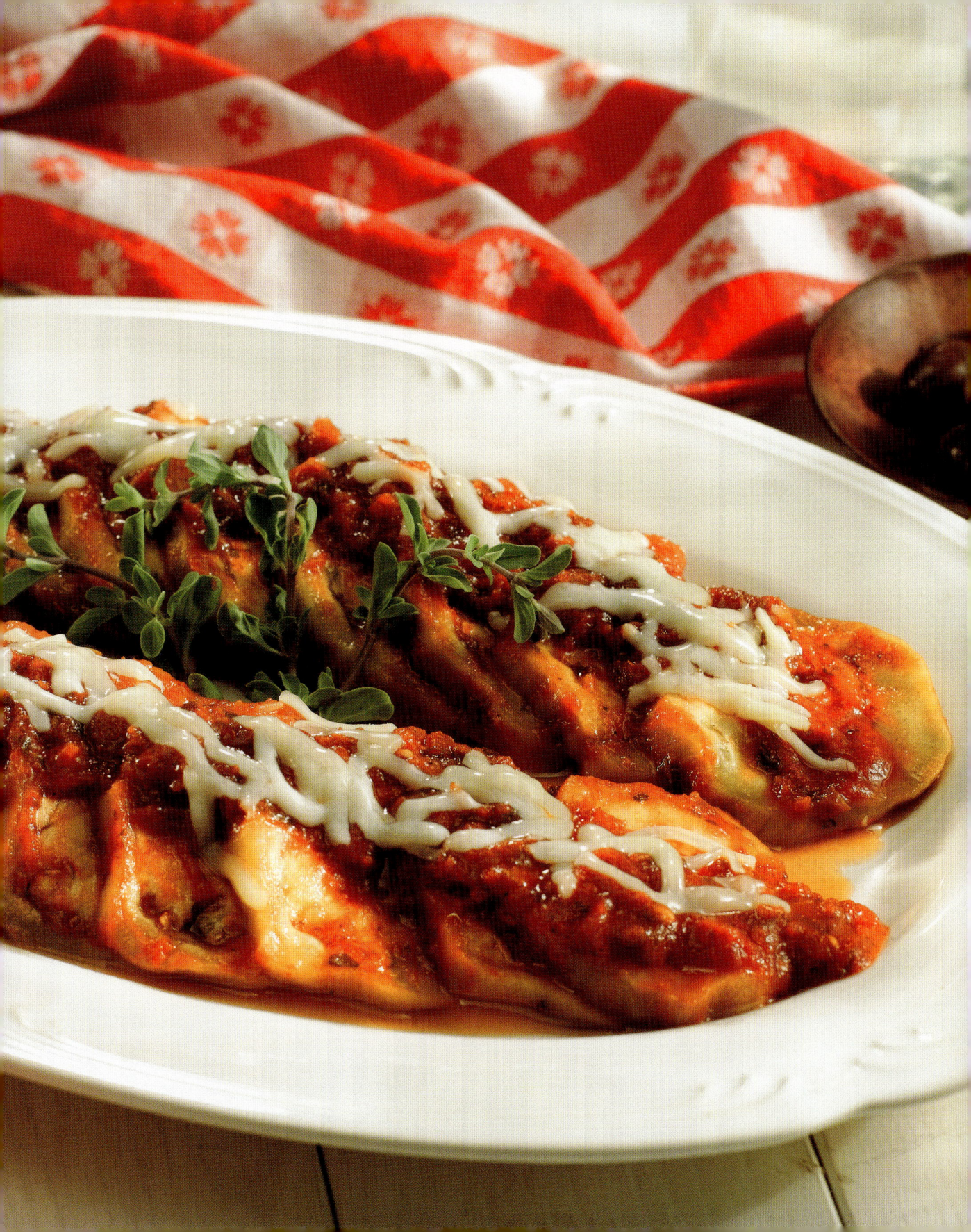

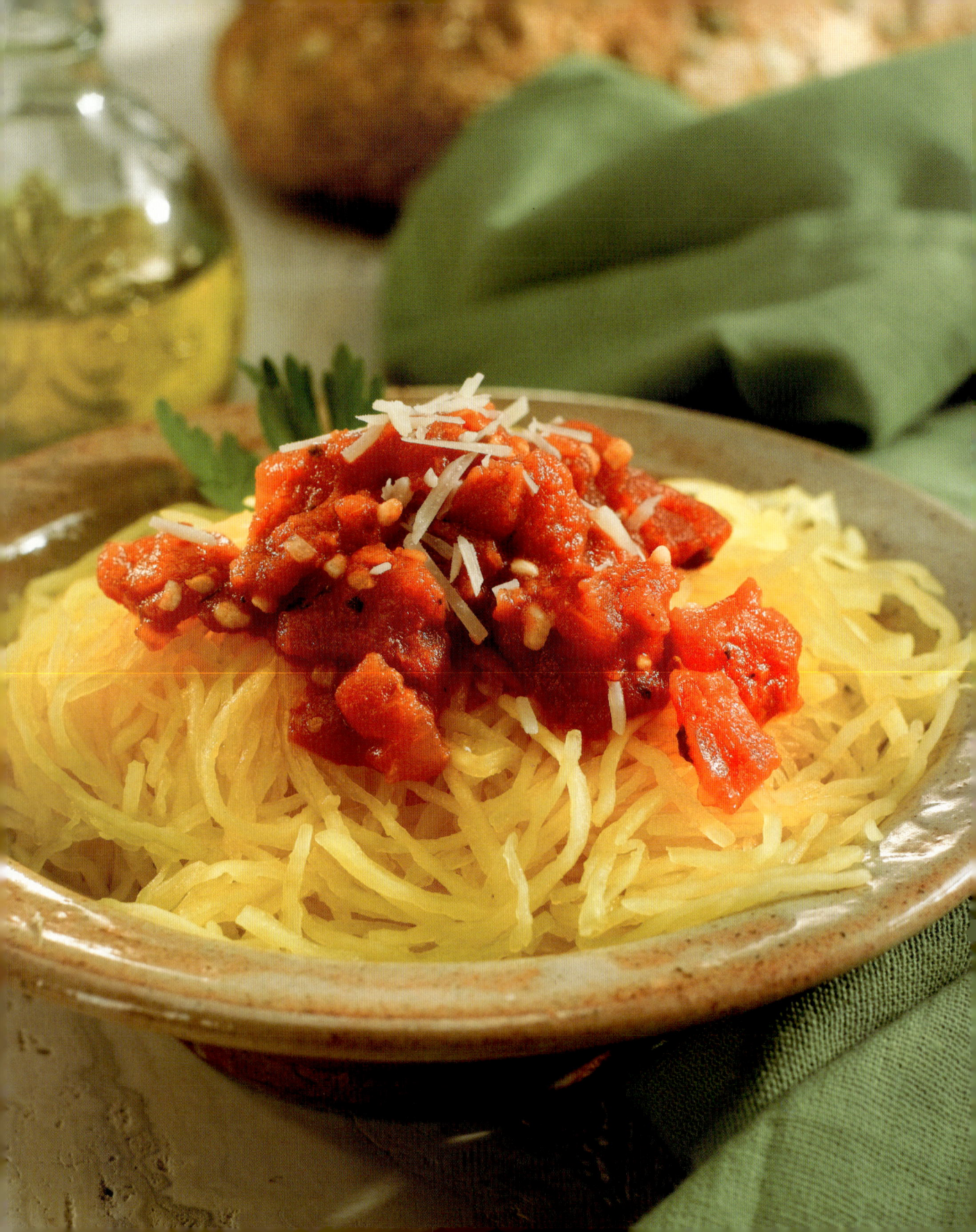

Spaghetti Squash with Pomodoro Sauce

TEXTURE: MECHANICAL SOFT

This is a wonderful substitute for pasta in a delicious sauce.

1 medium spaghetti squash (enough to yield 2 cups, or 310 g cooked)

1½ cups (570 ml) water

1 can (14⅛ ounces, or 415 g) diced tomatoes in juice, no salt added

2 cloves garlic, minced

6 tablespoons (3 ounces, or 90 ml) white wine or chicken broth or vegetable broth

½ teaspoon kosher salt

½ teaspoon ground white pepper

1 tablespoon (14 ml) extra-virgin olive oil

1 tablespoon (5 g) grated Parmesan cheese

Fresh parsley sprigs

—
Yield: Makes 4 (about ¾-cup) servings

Preheat the oven to 375° (190°C, or gas mark 5).

Cut the squash in half lengthwise and scrape out and discard the seeds. Place the halves in a baking dish, skin sides up. Add the water to the baking dish and bake about 40 minutes, until the squash will gently peel away from the skin with a fork.

In a 1- or 2-quart (1- or 2-L) saucepan, place the tomatoes with juice, garlic, wine or broth, salt, white pepper, and oil, cover, and bring to a simmer. Once a simmer is reached, remove the cover and continue cooking for 20 minutes.

For a smoother consistency, an emersion blender can be used to slightly puree the sauce.

Remove the cooked spaghetti squash by gently peeling away from the skin with a fork. Arrange in 1-cup (155 g) mounds on serving plates or in serving bowls as you would pasta and top with the sauce. Garnish with the cheese and parsley.

MARGARET'S NOTE

This delicious dish provides almost half of your vitamin C for the day. If you'd like to make a complete meal out of this, add about 3 ounces (85 g) shredded part-skim mozzarella cheese or shredded vegetarian (soy) cheese.

NUTRITIONAL ANALYSIS

EACH WITH: Calories: 96.47, Protein: 1.80 g, Carbs: 10.21 g, Total Fat: 4.01 g, Sat Fat: 0.69 g, Cholesterol: 0.25 mg, Sodium: 274.69 mg, Sugars: 4.29 g, Fiber: 2.09 g

Vegetarian Shepherd's Pie

TEXTURE: SOFT

Lentils make this dish high in fiber, hearty, and delicious.

1½ cups (290 g) green or brown lentils

1½ pounds (700 g) russet potatoes

3 tablespoons (45 g) light butter, divided

1 small yellow onion, diced (about ¾ cup, or 120 g)

½ cup (65 g) chopped carrot (about 1 medium)

1 medium celery rib, halved lengthwise and thinly sliced

2 cloves garlic, chopped

1 teaspoon salt

½ teaspoon black pepper

1 teaspoon dried basil

1 teaspoon dried oregano

1 teaspoon dried thyme

¼ teaspoon cayenne pepper (optional)

¼ cup (15 g) chopped fresh parsley

2 medium tomatoes, cored and diced

2 tablespoons (28 ml) soy milk, unsweetened

¾ cup (85 g) soy Cheddar cheese (optional)

½ teaspoon paprika

—

Yield: Makes 8 (about 1-cup) servings

In a bowl with water, soak the lentils for 30 minutes.

Peel and dice the potatoes into about 1-inch (2.5-cm) cubes. Place the potatoes in a 2½ -quart (2.5-L) saucepan with cold water to cover about 1 inch (2.5 cm) above the level of the potatoes.

Bring the potatoes to a boil and continue cooking for about 12 minutes, until the potatoes are tender throughout and will mash easily with a fork. Drain the potatoes in a colander and set aside.

In a 2-quart (2-L) saucepan, place the lentils with 3 cups (705 ml) of cold water and bring them to a boil. Reduce the heat to a simmer, loosely cover the pot, and continue cooking for about 30 minutes, or until all the liquid is absorbed and the lentils are tender.

Preheat the oven to 350°F (180°C, or gas mark 4). Coat a 2-quart (2-L) deep baking dish with cooking spray.

In a 9- or 10-inch (22.5- or 25-cm) skillet, melt 1 tablespoon (14 g) of the butter alternative over medium-high heat. Add the onion, carrots, celery, garlic, salt, pepper, basil, oregano, thyme, and cayenne pepper (if using) and sauté for about 5 minutes, until the carrots begin to soften, stirring occasionally. Add the parsley and tomatoes and continue to cook for about 3 minutes. Remove from the heat.

Mash the cooked lentils slightly with a large serving spoon and add them to the vegetable mixture, stirring just enough to incorporate. Spread the mixture evenly in the prepared baking dish and set aside.

Mash the potatoes together with 2 tablespoons (28 g) of the butter alternative, the soy milk, and soy cheese. Distribute the mashed potatoes

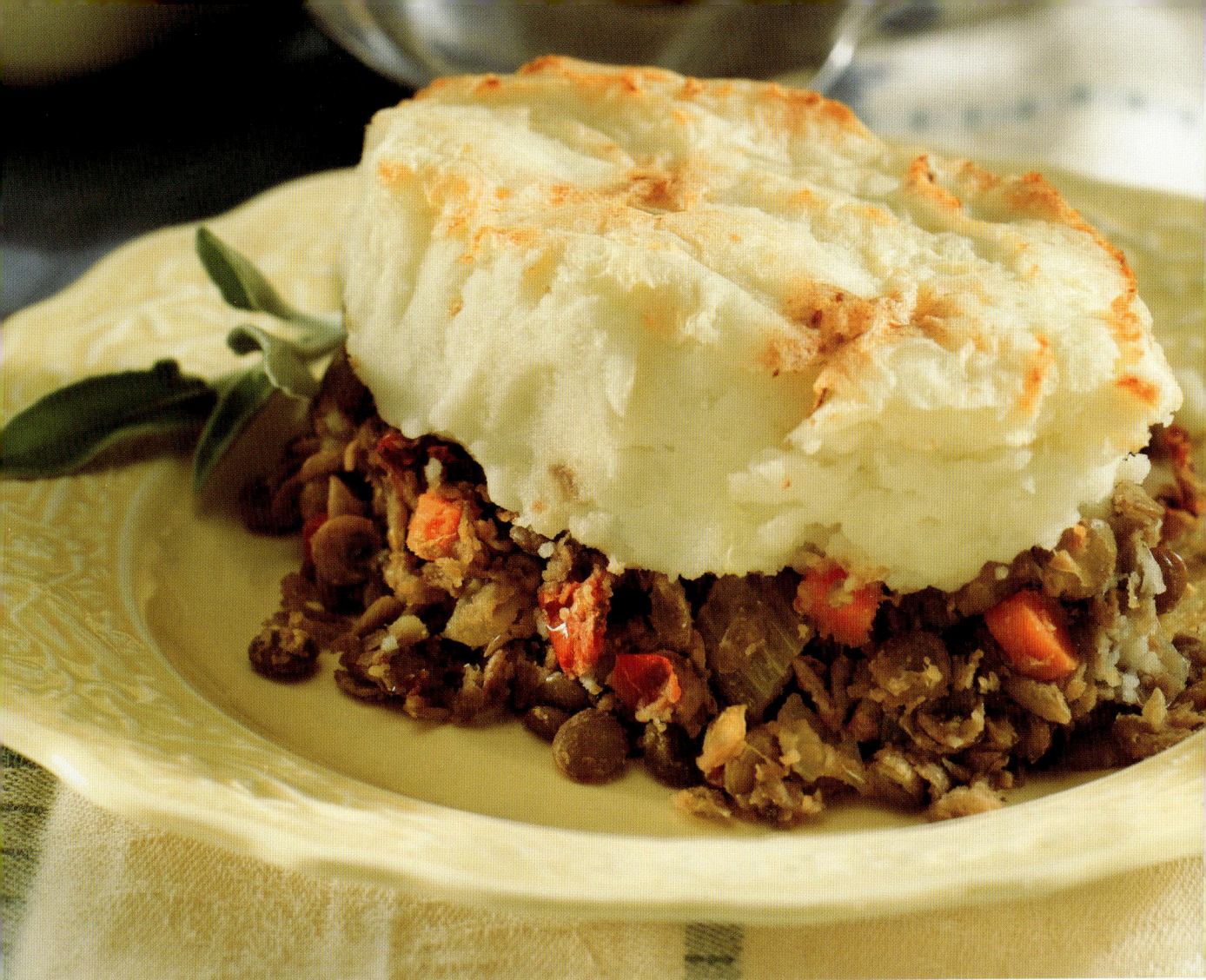

over the lentil-vegetable mixture and bake in the oven for 30 minutes, until the top appears golden brown. Serve hot and garnish with the paprika.

NUTRITIONAL ANALYSIS

EACH WITH: Calories: 235.36, Protein: 13.11 g, Carbs: 41.55 g, Total Fat: 3.06 g, Sat Fat: 0.49 g, Cholesterol: 0.00 mg, Sodium: 214.17 mg, Sugars: 5.04 g, Fiber: 14.63 g

MARGARET'S NOTE

You could add ¾ cup of soy or vegetarian cheese to this recipe. Add it while making the potato topping or grate it on top of the finished dish. Also, you could substitute adzuki beans or green or yellow split peas instead of all, or some, of the lentils.

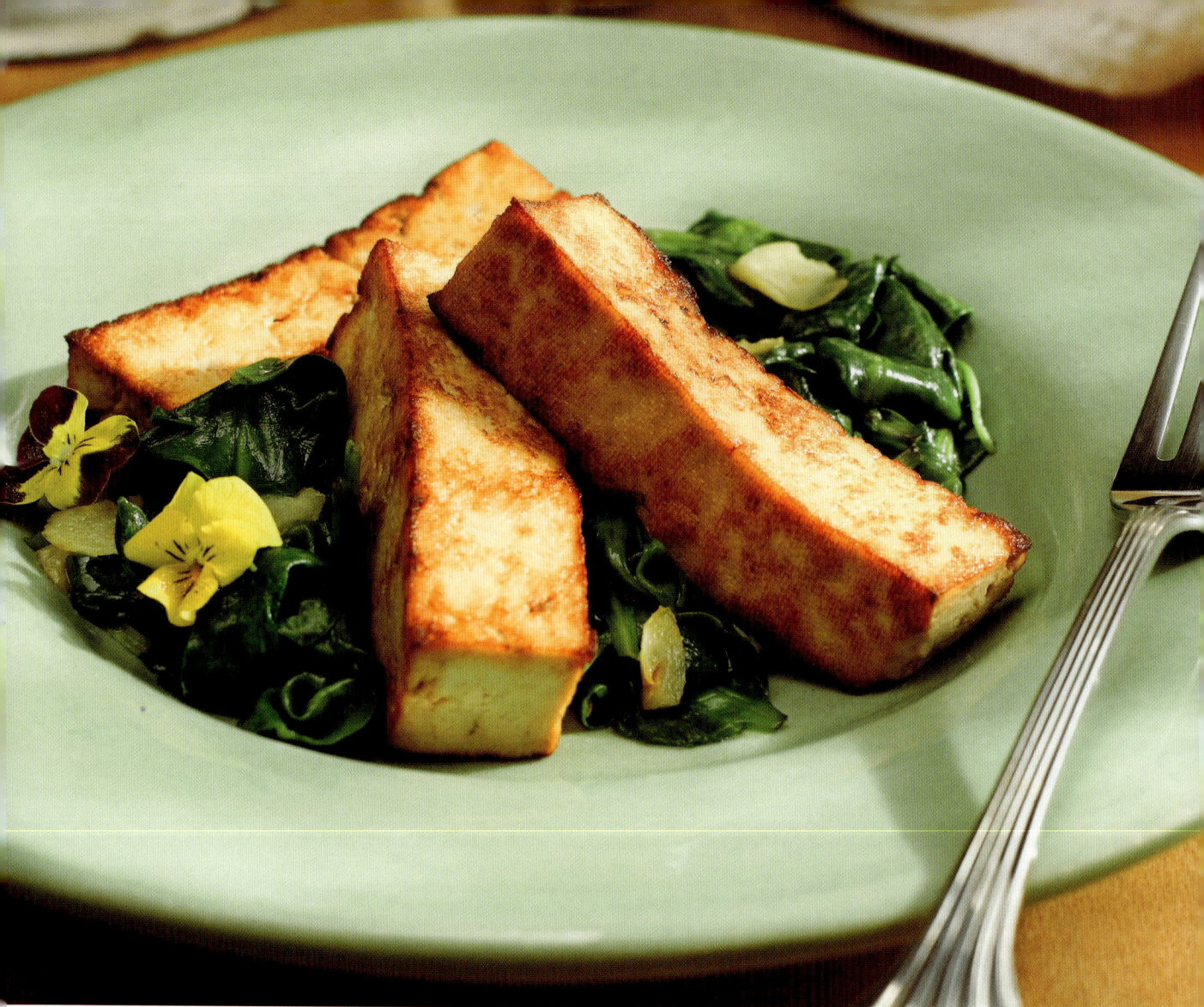

MARGARET'S NOTE

This dish is a bit higher in sodium than normally recommended (usually 700 milligrams or less per meal, for those who are salt-sensitive and/or need to watch sodium intake for blood pressure reasons), but it may be suitable for most people. If sodium is not an issue, you may add a bit of kosher salt to the spinach for added flavor. Also, you can increase the protein content of this dish by adding shredded soy cheese to the spinach. Another option is to toast about ⅛ to ¼ cup (12 to 25 g) of slivered almonds and sprinkle on top. This will add a bit more fat, but no cholesterol, and it will also increase the protein content.

Tasty Baked Tofu with Sautéed Spinach

TEXTURE: SOFT

Delicious vegetarian meals don't come easier than this.

2 tablespoons (28 ml) light soy sauce

⅛ teaspoon toasted sesame oil

2 tablespoons (28 ml) apple cider vinegar

1 clove garlic, minced

1 package (16 ounces, 455 g) firm tofu, drained and cut into cubes or cutlets

10 cups (200 g) fresh spinach

2 teaspoons extra-virgin olive oil

1 clove garlic, sliced into thin strips

Juice of 1 lemon

½ teaspoon black pepper

—

Yield: Makes 4 (about ½-cup) servings

In a 7- or 8-inch (17.5- or 20-cm) baking dish, place the soy sauce, sesame oil, vinegar, and minced garlic. Add the tofu. Marinate for 1 hour, turning the tofu once to expose all sides to the marinade.

Preheat the oven to 350°F (180°C, or gas mark 4).

Drain the excess marinade from the tofu and discard. Bake the tofu for approximately 30 minutes.

Meanwhile, wash, drain, and chop the spinach into 1-inch (2.5-cm) strips. (If using baby spinach, leave it in whole leaves.) Pat the spinach dry with a paper towel.

In an 8-inch (20-cm) skillet, heat the oil over medium heat. Add the sliced garlic and sauté just enough to sweat the garlic. (Do not brown.) Add the spinach, lemon juice, and pepper. Cook for about 4 to 6 minutes, stirring often, until the spinach is tender. Place the spinach on a serving dish and top with the tofu.

NUTRITIONAL ANALYSIS

EACH WITH: Calories: 224.85, Protein: 23.89 g, Carbs: 19.95 g, Total Fat: 5.83 g, Sat Fat: 0.33 g, Cholesterol: 0.00 mg, Sodium: 1492.84 mg, Sugars: 1.56 g, Fiber: 10.09 g

About the Authors

Margaret Furtado, M.S., R.D., L.D.N., R.Y.T., is a registered and licensed dietitian with over twenty years of clinical experience, including approximately ten years in medical and surgical weight loss, and is also a registered yoga teacher. She is currently seeing patients in the outpatient setting as a clinical dietitian specialist at the Johns Hopkins Center for Bariatric Surgery, in Baltimore, Maryland, including pre- and postop gastric banding, sleeve, gastric bypass and D/S patients. Prior to this position, Ms. Furtado worked at Massachusetts General Hospital's Weight Center and Tufts Medical Center's Weight and Wellness Center. She earned her master's degree in nutrition and dietetics at Florida International University, in Miami, and her bachelor of science degree in nutrition and dietetics from the University of Rhode Island. Ms. Furtado was a coauthor on the American Society for Metabolic and Bariatric Surgery's bariatric nutrition guideline paper, and lectures internationally on issues pertaining to nutrition and weight-loss surgery. In December 2009, her second book, The Complete Idiot's Guide to Eating Well After Weight Loss Surgery was released, and she has also authored a mini-ebook on preparing for bariatric surgery.

Lynette Schultz, chef, L.R.C.P., R.T., received her culinary training at various venues around the Seattle area. She currently works as a guest chef at Hedgebrook, a retreat for women writers near her home on Whidbey Island, Washington, and as a licensed respiratory care practitioner at Whidbey General Hospital.

Chef Joseph Ewing, holds a bachelor of science degree in culinary nutrition and an associate of science degree in culinary arts from Johnson & Wales University. He is the coauthor, with Margaret Furtado, M.S., R.D., L.D.N., R.Y.T., of The Complete Idiot's Guide to Eating Well after Weight Loss Surgery. Joseph began his culinary career in catering, and then later obtained a cooking position in a restaurant in his hometown of Easton, Maryland. He was awarded first place in the state of Maryland SkillsUSA National Culinary Arts Contest. In nearly a decade of culinary experience ranging from restaurant work, catering, and as a personal chef, Chef Ewing has worked and studied under a number of talented chefs and developed a great deal of knowledge and skill in the craft. He is currently studying to become a registered dietitian through the University of Maryland Eastern Shore Dietetic Internship Program.

Index